THE JAYNES LEGACY

SHINING NEW LIGHT THROUGH THE CRACKS OF THE BICAMERAL MIND

Lawrence Wile

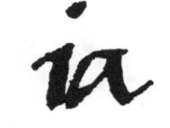

imprint-academic.com

Copyright © Lawrence Wile, 2018

The moral rights of the authors have been asserted.
No part of this publication may be reproduced in any form
without permission, except for the quotation of brief passages
in criticism and discussion.

Published in the UK by
Imprint Academic, PO Box 200, Exeter EX5 5YX, UK

Distributed in the USA by
Ingram Book Company,
One Ingram Blvd., La Vergne, TN 37086, USA

ISBN 9781845409227

A CIP catalogue record for this book is available from the
British Library and US Library of Congress

Contents

Introduction	1
One: *The Origins of Consciousness in the Breakdown of the Bicameral Mind*: A Synopsis	5
Two: Origins of *The Origins of Consciousness in the Breakdown of the Bicameral Mind*	35
Three: Assessment	41
Four: Reissner's Fiber	76
Five: Is Science a Vestige of the Search for Lost Hallucinatory Gods?	94
Six: Reissner's Fiber, the "Subtle Anatomy," and the Devil	122
Seven: Is the Old Testament an Account of the Breakdown of the Bicameral Mind?	159
Eight: The Legacy of Julian Jaynes: Shining New Light Through the Cracks in the Bicameral Mind	170
Bibliography	186
Index	192

Introduction

Julian Jaynes's 1976 book, *The Origins of Consciousness in the Breakdown of the Bicameral Mind*, continues to arouse an unsettling ambivalence. Richard Dawkins called it "either complete rubbish or a work of consummate genius, nothing in between." It is, in my opinion, "complete rubbish" because Jaynes's analysis of consciousness contravenes logic and self-evident psychological truths. The bicameral mind as the orchestrator of a hierarchical theocracy of nonconscious individuals via auditory hallucinations is a phantasm. The dating of the origin of consciousness contradicts archeological and literary evidence. The theory contributes nothing toward explaining why some physical states are conscious while others are not because the nonconscious bicameral brain is neurophysiologically equivalent to the conscious brain.

On the flip side it is, in my opinion, a work of "consummate genius" because it inspires us to reinterpret humankind's earliest religious traditions and texts in ways that might shine light on the "very suspicious totem of evolutionary mythology" which has dissuaded us from our intuition that consciousness has not evolved continuously and gradually from worms to man. The evolution of consciousness took a qualitative leap during the era of *Homo sapiens*. Furthermore, Jaynes's interpretation of our earliest religious texts as factual accounts based on states of consciousness radically different from our own inspires us to explore new neuropsychological interpretations of religion.

However, while Jaynes boldly challenges evolutionary theory's axiom that consciousness has always evolved continuously and gradually, he worships at the altar of its axiom that consciousness emerged from nonconscious physical reactions. The difference between Jaynes's emergentism and conventional emergentism is that Jaynes dates the emergence of consciousness at 1000 BC while conventional emergentism places the date at 500 million BC, or perhaps much earlier, to the level of organization of the first single-celled organisms. According to Jaynes, until 1000 BC, hallucinations, poetry, and civilizations were merely nonconscious physical reactivity.

Instead of clarifying the mechanisms and dates of the emergence of consciousness, Jaynes inadvertently highlights the vacuity of consciousness as an emergent phenomenon. His magnificent failure to explain the origin of consciousness is not due solely to the preposterous dating of the emergence of consciousness at 1000 BC, but to the principle of emergentism itself. An unintended part of Jaynes's legacy, therefore, is the inspiration to re-examine emergentism.

My book, *The Jaynes Legacy: Shining New Light Through the Cracks of the Bicameral Mind*, explores the possibility that consciousness pre-existed matter. Consciousness is coeternal with the initial singularity that gave rise to spacetime. This characterization of consciousness is consistent with the infinite regress of the consciousness of consciousness and the consciousness of the consciousness of consciousness and so on, free will, and the capacity of human consciousness to discover natural laws and mathematical truths.

Consciousness began its relationship with physical reality during the leap from "nothing" to "something" 13.8 billion years ago. More than ten billion years later, pockets of negentropy fueled by the sun evolved into the first living cells on earth. Nanoengineered microtubules constituting cilia, centrioles, mitotic spindles, and neuronal cytoskeletons served as functional interfaces with the "nothingness" of the eternal vacuum wherein virtual particles and antiparticles are created and annihilated in the zero-point field.

Five hundred million years ago, during the Cambrian explosion, glycoproteins in the fluid-filled neurocele of protovertebrates aggregated around a one-dimensional thread to form an evolutionarily persistent, little known, threadlike structure called Reissner's fiber. This macroscopic structure greatly amplified quantum coherences achieved by microtubules. The relationship between consciousness and physical reality was thereby greatly strengthened.

One hundred thousand yeas ago, consciousness took another leap when the analog language of screeches and howls transformed into a digital infinity. The idea of physical objects independent of the perceptions that gave rise to them brought humankind to the threshold of the road of science and the unification of experience into a rational system. Coinciding with this leap of consciousness was the epigenetically induced perinatal involution of Reissner's fiber in humans.

Over the course of thousands of generations, the dynamic self-referential, digital web of language that began with nouns directly connected to the triggerings of sensory neurons progressed toward greater and greater conceptual unity. About 6,000 yeas ago, it converged upon its center. Humankind transcended itself and contemplated its origins, meaning, and ultimate destiny. But, like the self-referential point of an Escher drawing, the words used to represent the center of the web—Brahman, Tao, and God—embraced contradictions and reflected the ineffable.

Consistent with Jaynes's interpretation of religious texts as factual accounts based on a mentality radically different from our own, I propose that descriptions of the "subtle anatomy" from humankind's earliest mystical traditions—the *nadis* and *chakras* of yoga, the meridians and vessels of acupuncture as applied Taoism, and the *Sephirot* of Kabbalah—are based on interoceptions of Reissner's fiber by a few rare individuals for whom the fiber persisted into adulthood. We currently know the subtlest activities of the fiber as mathematical abstractions representing transtemporal, multidimensional realities and a hierarchy of infinites. We are denied direct consciousness of what is represented by these abstractions, because, according to quantum theory, they are only there when no one is looking. Quantum orthodoxy, therefore, denies realism. I propose that the quantum world is real and that Reissner's fiber as a macroscopic quantum system allows the direct supersensory consciousness of it.

The authors of our earliest religious texts had access to supersensory perceptions mediated by Reissner's fiber, but their teachings, out of necessity, were communicated in the digital infinity of language that had separated humankind's consciousness from its eternal source. Humankind moved further and further from knowledge based on supersensory perceptions based on the fiber. By the sixth century BC, the era of prophecy, the era of direct consciousness of the eternal source of consciousness ended. But beneath the dust of fallen Babel lies the blueprint for a unified neurocosmology organized around Reissner's fiber, a roadmap to transcendence and salvation. Now, 6,000 years after the original convergence of the web of language upon its center was integrated with interoceptions of Reissner's fiber, a new mathematically precise language and technological enhancements of our sensory experience is bringing us to the threshold of a higher integration in which interoceptions are synthesized with exteroceptions of the reborn fiber at the limit of objectivity.

My proposed neurocosmology organized around Reissner's fiber is currently an insubstantial web of parallels between ancient mystical traditions and modern science, scientific speculation, preliminary evidence of evanescent quantum biophysical effects, and the fiber's associations with neural circuits involved with altered states of consciousness. Reissner's fiber seen through the current lens of science is a morphogenetic structure that typically involutes during late human fetal development and might be involved in the pathogenesis of hydrocephalus, the detoxification of the spinal fluid, or possibly in the promotion of neurogenesis in adults to repair the effects of degenerative and traumatic brain disease. However, now, for the first time in history, we have the tools to control the epigenetic factors responsible for the fiber's typical involution and regenerate it. New technologies could provide feedback of the fiber's activity at the limits of objectivity—the quantum level—and thereby create the opportunity of controlling and amplifying its possible quantum effects. We can begin a journey along an ancient, forgotten, broken, strategically located neural circuit to explore the frontiers of consciousness. A journey into the unknown.

One

The Origins of Consciousness in the Breakdown of the Bicameral Mind
A Synopsis

Julian Jaynes's notion that humans were not conscious until 3,000 years ago continues to entice and perplex us. "If our reasonings have been correct," he tells us, "it is perfectly possible that there could have existed a race of men who spoke, judged, reasoned, solved problems, indeed did most of the things that we do, but were not conscious at all." What, then, *is* consciousness? What explains its recent origin?

Consciousness, according to Jaynes, is a dynamic web of metaphors weaving itself within an introspectable mind-space. It weaves not only the stuff of consciousness but also the weaver, an "analog 'I'". Before the origin of consciousness, a pre-conscious "bicameral mind" fed voices from Wernicke's area of the right cerebral hemisphere to the left hemisphere via the anterior commissure. These auditory hallucinations, perceived as gods, were unconsciously obeyed as neural commands. About three thousand years ago, natural disasters, and the stresses and complexities of growing societies, overwhelmed the fragile bicameral order. It broke down. From its remains, an introspectable mind-space emerged which told the tale of its breakdown and rebirth. Vestiges of the bicameral origins of consciousness persist as auditory hallucinations heard by schizophrenics and the longing for lost gods.

Jaynes illustrates his definition of consciousness with a line from a poem: "my love is like a tinsmith's scoop, sunk past its gleam in the meal bin." Here, as interpreted by Jaynes, we find "the enduring careful shape and hidden shiningness and holdingness of a lasting love deep in the heavy manipulable softness of mounding time, the whole simulating (and so paraphranding[1]) sexual intercourse from a male point of view." "Love," Jaynes declares, "has not such properties except as we generate them by metaphor. Of such poetry is consciousness made."

Having concluded that poetry is the stuff of consciousness, Jaynes lures the reader to follow him on his journey to this conclusion with a poetic evocation of the tension between mind and matter, subject and object, soul and body: "O, WHAT A WORLD of unseen visions and heard silences, this unsubstantial country of the mind!" Consciousness, for Jaynes, is a wondrous, paradoxical, mysterious, secret, inner kingdom. Matter, objects, and bodies, for Jaynes, constitute "the ordered array of nature that somehow surrounds and engulfs this core of knowing." Consciousness is a "fabric of fancy." Brains, like "trees, grass, tables, oceans, hands, stars," are part of "handable, standable, kickable reality." Jaynes thus locates the essential core of the problem of consciousness in the nature of consciousness rather than matter.

The theory of evolution, according to Jaynes, transformed the mind–body problem into the problem of when consciousness evolved from "mere matter." Therefore, he begins his analysis with a review of what believes to be the most important modern evolutionary solutions to the problem of consciousness. He concludes that they are misguided.

Consciousness as a Property of Matter

First, Jaynes looks at "consciousness as a property of matter." According to his analysis, this solution to the riddle of consciousness proposes that consciousness stretches back to prebiotic matter. The relationship between mind and matter is not fundamentally different from the relationship between a tree and the ground in which it is rooted or the gravitational relationship between celestial bodies. Historically, Alexander's theory of comprence and Whitehead's theory of prehension laid the groundwork for this view, which flourished in the first quarter of the twentieth century as a type of monism known as Neo-realism. Its attractiveness was based on the "astonishing success of particle physics." Beneath the subtle, complex arguments of the Neo-

---

[1] "Paraphranding" is a neologism coined by Jaynes to describe the self-referential process of expanding metaphors. A paraphrand is one of four neologisms employed by Jaynes to describe the origination of conscious from the development of metaphors. The first is a "metaphier," a familiar direct sensory percept that conveys some meaning beyond its literal one, thereby creating a "metaphrand." A "paraphier" of a metaphrand maps onto the metaphrand creating deeper layers of meaning and thus becomes the metaphrand's paraphrand.

realists of the early twentieth century, he writes, lies the proposition that the interaction between a piece of chalk dropped onto a table differs only in complexity from conscious perception and knowing. This theory fails because it explains only the interaction between matter and its environment and omits our introspectable, subjective experience. Modern physics, with its dissolving of matter into unvisualizable, mathematical abstractions, merely created the illusion of a bridge between mind and matter.

Consciousness as a Property of Protoplasm

"Consciousness is a property of protoplasm" is a second failed solution to the mind–body problem. While amoebas seeking food and paramecia avoiding prey seem to be exhibiting conscious, intelligent behaviors, their behaviors are actually explained by physical chemistry, not introspective psychology. We see a worm wriggling on an angler's hook and project feelings of agony. However, upon further examination we note that the lower half of a cut worm writhes even more that the upper half with its primitive brain. The agony we see is our own, not the worm's. The wriggling is caused by a release of motor neurons from their cephalic inhibition.

Consciousness as Learning

"Consciousness as learning" is a third failed solution that owes its attractiveness to "a kind of huge historical neurosis" that resulted from its championing by prestigious scientists during the eighteenth and nineteenth centuries. They erroneously believed that consciousness is a place inhabited by ideas and sensations. Therefore, learning and consciousness became confused and conflated with the muddled notion of experience.

Theories of consciousness as a property of matter or protoplasm, or as learning, all share the assumption that consciousness evolved gradually and continuously from random genetic variation and natural selection. This "continuity hypothesis of Darwin," Jaynes writes, "is a very suspicious totem of evolutionary mythology." With poetic eloquence Jaynes urges us to ponder "The yearning for certainty which grails the scientist, the aching beauty which harasses the artist, the sweet thorn of justice which fierces the rebel from the eases of life, or the thrill of exultation with which we hear true acts of that now difficult virtue of courage, of hopeless suffering." "Are these really derivable from matter … Or even continuous with the idiot hierarchies of speechless apes?" he asks. Human conscious, he believes, exploded in a new direction thousands of years ago creating an awesome chasm that separates us from other mammals.

Consciousness as a Metaphysical Imposition

Alfred Russel Wallace, co-discoverer of the theory of evolution through natural selection, engaged in a fierce struggle with Darwin about the continuity of the evolution of consciousness. Darwin's final book, published a year before his death, investigated how far earthworms "acted consciously and how much mental power they displayed." Based on his observations that a worm's tendency to "dash like a rabbit into its burrow" when suddenly illuminated could be modified, he concluded that this behavior was not merely a reflex. He further noted that worms exhibit "mental qualities" when they plug up their burrows. They are able to judge how to best drag an object and therefore "deserve to be called intelligent, for they then act in nearly the same manner as a man under similar circumstances." Jaynes wrote that the marvelous continuity of life that Darwin had discovered blinded him to the "terrifying and absolute" discontinuity of human consciousness. Darwin "clouded the problem with naiveté."

Wallace believed that what Jaynes refers to as a "metaphysical imposition" was responsible for endowing humankind with its unique capacities. This belief led Wallace to attend séances and search for answers from Spiritualists. He thereby stepped outside the boundaries of the "scientific Establishment." He was ostracized. He had stepped outside "the rules of natural science." "And that indeed was the problem," Jaynes writes, "how to explain consciousness in terms of natural science alone." Thus, "consciousness as a metaphysical imposition" becomes the fourth theory that Jaynes rejects as a solution to the mind–body problem.

The Helpless Spectator Theory

The backlash against metaphysical explanations of consciousness led to increasingly materialist theories. Among them is the fifth solution rejected by Jaynes, the "helpless spectator theory," according to which consciousness is a mere epiphenomenon that does nothing. We are, according to this theory, in the words of Thomas Huxley, "Darwin's bulldog," "conscious automatons" whose volitions are merely symbols of brain states. Jaynes rejects Huxley's characterization of humans and subscribes to William James's common-sense defense of free will: "It is just inconceivable that consciousness should have nothing to do."

Emergent Evolution

The sixth theory rejected by Jaynes is "emergent evolution." This theory elevated consciousness from its untenable position as a "helpless spectator" and replaced "metaphysical impositions" as the explanation of the evolutionary discontinuities of life and consciousness.

The basic idea of emergentism is that consciousness is not derivable from the constituent parts of the system from which it emerged. Its main idea, according to Jaynes, is a metaphor: just as wetness is underivable from the properties of hydrogen and oxygen, so too is consciousness underivable from the properties of neurons. Jaynes advocates strong emergence. The emergent level has new downward causal properties.

Emergentism captured the imagination of biologists and neurologists who had felt compelled to suppress observed results not discovered nor expected from work on non-living systems. Consciousness was restored to its "throne as the governor of behavior."

Jaynes initially enthusiastically embraced emergent evolution. It liberated biology from physics and chemistry. However, eventually, he came to see emergent evolution as mere hand-waving, a license for "vacuous generalities." The theory does not answer the questions of when consciousness emerged, in what species it emerged, or what kind of nervous system is necessary for its emergence.

Behaviorism

While enthusiasm for emergent evolution was building, another solution to the problem of consciousness was creating a robust experimental program to conquer the field of psychology. The seventh theory explored and rejected by Jaynes is behaviorism. It attempted to solve the problem of consciousness with the startling doctrine that consciousness doesn't exist at all.

Jaynes traces the origins of behaviorism to eighteenth-century objectivism and actionism. John B. Watson coined the term behaviorism in 1913 when he proposed to make psychology a "purely objective experimental branch of natural science" that is independent of introspection or interpretations based on consciousness. "The behaviorist," Watson declared, "in his efforts to get a unitary scheme of animal response, recognizes no dividing line between man and brute."

Behaviorism dominated psychology from about 1920 to 1960. Jaynes traces its ascendance to a longing to extricate psychology from the vagueness and obscurity of philosophy and the desire to ground psychology in objective facts. Psychology would have a fresh start!

Exhilarated by the "gleaming stainless-steel promise of reducing all conduct to a handful of reflexes and conditional response," behaviorists conquered academic psychology. The effete opposition of Titchenerian introspectionism faded away. Those interested in the problem of consciousness were "forcibly excluded from academia" and texts "tried to smother the unwanted problem from student view."

Jaynes confesses that, having been a part of behaviorism, it was not what a seemed. It was not a theory. It was method practiced by hypocrites: "Nobody really believed he was not conscious." However, as Jaynes notes, the rigorous methods of behaviorism and its grounding in conditioned neural responses played an important role in sweeping out the ghosts of empty metaphysical speculations and thereby creating a new playing field.

Consciousness as the Reticular Activating System

The eighth theory rejected by Jaynes is "consciousness as the reticular activating system." This theory, which, at the time of Jaynes's writings, was a recently proposed plausible neural substrate of consciousness, is based on neurophysiological data that show that this evolutionary ancient network of nerves regulates attention and the transition between wakefulness and sleep. Jaynes dismissively puts this proposal on the historical spectrum of "fervent if often superficial" searches for the physical seat of consciousness such as Descartes' misguided speculation that the pineal gland is the seat of the soul. Furthermore, because Jaynes identifies consciousness with language, he rejects the idea that the reticular activating system, which evolved hundreds of millions of years ago, can provide the answer to the problem of consciousness and its origins.

Having rejected "consciousness as the reticular activating system" as the solution to the problem of consciousness, Jaynes goes further and contends that neuroscientists who seek to translate psychological phenomena into neurophysiology are following a "delusional line of reasoning." From his observation that, even we if we knew the complete wiring diagram of the nervous system, every synapse, and every neurotransmitter, "we could still never—*not ever*—from knowledge of the brain alone know if that brain contained a consciousness like our own," Jaynes concludes that we must therefore start at the top. We must first be clear about our conception of consciousness before entering the world of neuroscience.

Jaynes believes that what appear to most of us as self-evident truths about consciousness are false. We must sweep away those false ideas to arrive at a clear conception of consciousness.

The Consciousness of Consciousness

Jaynes asserts that, contrary to what most of us think, consciousness of consciousness is not what consciousness is. Our awareness of our selves, of our sensations, moods, thoughts, memories, and volitions, has been masquerading as consciousness for centuries. All these mental phenomena actually operate in the unconscious depths of the mind.

Jaynes first argues that much of what we regard as consciousness is actually mere reactivity. While sitting against a tree, for example, we are constantly, unconsciously, reacting to the tree, the ground, and our own posture. If we wish to walk, we will unconsciously rise from the ground to do so. Jaynes observes that while he is writing he is conscious only of what he is trying to say and whether or not he is communicating clearly. The feel of the pencil in his hand and of the writing pad between his knees involves only unconscious reactivity. If a bird outside his window should fly toward the horizon and he should turn and follow its flight, this would similarly involve only unconscious reactivity.

Our visual system is constantly performing tasks unconsciously to create perceptual continuity amidst neuronal flickerings and retinal shifts. We adjust our perception of depth and contrast unconsciously. We unconsciously fill in the two-millimeter blind spot on the nasal side of the retina. Jaynes analogizes consciousness searching its mental life with a flashlight searching a dark room, looking for something that does not have any light shining upon it. The flashlight, according to Jaynes, would conclude that there is light everywhere, just as consciousness seems to pervade all mentality.

The pianist who loses himself in rapturous ecstasy, the athlete who relies on muscle memory ingrained by hours of practice, or the experienced driver who responds instinctively to changing road conditions are not conscious. Not only is consciousness unnecessary for the performance of complex activities, it can be detrimental. Were a pianist to become conscious of the flexions of his fingers as they fluidly fly across the keys he would revert to the novice consciously reading and counting every note.

Consciousness is Not a Copy of Experience

After arguing that consciousness is far less extensive than most of us think, Jaynes asserts that the commonly held notion that consciousness is a copy of experience is confused. Our minds do not function like cameras, recording and storing sensory experience. To illustrate this point, Jaynes asks the reader to recall the following: which finger is the second longest? Is it the red or green light that is on the top of a traffic light? Which letters are associated with which letters on a telephone keyboard? What are the objects behind you in the familiar room? Although many of us would be surprised about how little we could recall if those familiar objects were rearranged, we would immediately recognize that something had changed. We *knew* all along, but were not conscious of knowing.

To further illustrate the point that consciousness is not a copy of experience, Jaynes asks readers to recall themselves swimming. Typically, we *see* ourselves swimming, something we have never observed at all. We recall very little of the feel of the water, of the extent our eyes were under water, or the turning of our head to breathe. Our conscious recall is an invention, not a copy of experience.

Consciousness Not Necessary for Concepts

Next, Jaynes argues that consciousness is not necessary for concepts. To make this point, he disputes the conclusion drawn by the nineteenth-century philologist and Vedic scholar Max Muller: "No one ever saw a tree, but only this or that fir tree, or oak tree, or apple tree ... Tree therefore, is a concept, and as such can never be seen or perceived by the senses." According to Jaynes, Muller confused what one knows about the object and the object itself. "Every weary wayfarer after miles under the hot sun has seen a tree," writes Jaynes. The bee has a concept of a flower, an eagle of a cliff, and a nesting bird of a crotch of an upper tree branch. "Concepts are simply classes of behaviorally equivalent things," that do not become elements of consciousness until they are represented by language.

Consciousness Not Necessary for Learning

Further, Jaynes presents evidence to show that consciousness is not necessary for learning. Jaynes first shows that learning as Pavlovian conditioning, or other types of associative learning, occurs unconsciously. For example, if a song is played while one is eating a delicious meal, that song will sound more pleasant the next time it is heard. Conscious awareness of the contingency between food and the song eliminates the conditioned learning; just as conscious thought impedes the performances of musicians, athletes, and orators. Not only are conditioned responses learned unconsciously, but goal oriented behaviors and complex motor skills are as well. Jaynes supports this contention with results from an experiment on subjects whose thumbs were attached to electrodes that sent signals that diminished an unpleasant noise when an imperceptible muscle twitch occurred. The subject unconsciously learned to increase their twitching. Thus, Jaynes concludes that "learning of signals, skills or solutions" occurs without consciousness.

Consciousness Not Necessary for Thinking

Next, Jaynes presents evidence to show that consciousness is not necessary for thinking. He invites the reader to hold two unequal objects, such as unequally filled glasses of water, and, with half-closed eyes, judge which one is heavier. While we would feel the texture and temperature of the glass, its protuberances, and the downward pull against our skin, we will not be conscious of judging which of the glasses is heavier, Jaynes avers. To support this contention, Jaynes cites a similar experiment performed in 1901 by the psychologist Karl Marbe. He reported that his experimental subjects were not conscious of the process of judging which of two unequal weights was greater. Just as the Michelson-Morley experiment disproved the ether, writes Jaynes, the Marbe experiment showed that "judging, the supposed hallmark of consciousness did not exist in consciousness at all."

To counter the argument that the judging involved in Marbe's experiments happened so fast that the subjects forget it, Jaynes points to experiments performed a few years later by H.J. Watt. He presented his subjects with nouns printed on cards and asked them to verbally associate the noun with another word as quickly as possible. The responses were not free associations, but were constrained by prior instructions. The subject might be instructed to give a part of the object. Oak might elicit the response acorn, for example. The subjects were then asked to introspect the various stages involved in the process; instruction, presentation of the card, search for a reply, and verbal response. Contrary to expectations, the subjects reported that the period during which they searched for an association was introspectively blank.

Drawing on the results from these experiments, Jaynes shows that other mental tasks such as finding the next figure in a series of alternating circles and triangles, or finding specific words or phrases as we speak, are performed unconsciously. The important part of these tasks is the instruction given prior to such mental tasks that allows the subsequent mental processes to occur automatically. Therefore, Jaynes concludes, thinking is not conscious.

Consciousness Not Necessary for Reason

Next, Jaynes elevates reason above thinking in general, because it follows the ideal of logic. However, like thinking, reason does not, according to Jaynes, require consciousness. Logic is the science of justifying our unconscious reasoning.

Jaynes's line of reasoning starts with the assertion that "[c]hoosing paths, words, notes, the perceptual corrections in size and color constancies" are all primitive forms of reasoning that operate outside consciousness. A more standard form of reasoning, the inference from the observation of one piece of wood floating in a pond that a new piece of wood will float in another pond occurs with no conscious deliberation. Such reasoning is hardwired into the nervous system of all higher vertebrates. It is not a part of the structure of consciousness.

Reasoning that is more complex occurs continuously. We generalize from particulars. We reach conclusions from past experiences without conscious reflection. We infer motives of others and assess their character as a result of unconscious neural programs.

To counter the reader's presumed protest that the highest flights of intellectual thought require conscious induction and deduction, Jaynes cites examples of sudden insights by great scientists and mathematicians. Their great insights sprang mysteriously from the depths of the unconscious. Helmholtz recalled that his flashes of insight "often enough crept quietly into my thinking without my suspecting their importance ... in other cases they arrived suddenly, without any effort on my part ... they liked especially to make their appearance while I was taking an easy walk over the wooded hills in sunny weather!" Gauss reported that the solution to a mathematical proof that had eluded his conscious efforts for years appeared, "like a sudden flash of lightning, the riddle happened to be solved. I myself cannot say what was the conducting thread which connected what I previously knew with what made my success possible." Poincaré described how he made a complex mathematical discovery while on a geological excursion: "The incidents of the journey made me forget my mathematical work. Having reached Coutances, we entered an omnibus to go some place or other. At the moment when I put my foot on the step, the idea came to me, without anything in my former thoughts seeming to have paved the way for it, the transformation I had used to define the Fuchsian functions were identical with those of non-Euclidean geometry!" From these examples, Jaynes concludes that there are three stages involved in creative thought: conscious thought, unconscious incubation, and illumination that is later justified by logic. While the period of preparation involves conscious attention, the actual reasoning, Jaynes contends, is the "dark leap into discovery" that "has no representation in consciousness."

The Location of Consciousness

After having dismissed consciousness of consciousness, consciousness as a copy of experience, concepts, learning, thinking, and reasoning from the realm of consciousness, Jaynes presents the case that consciousness is not in our heads. He leaves this argument for last because it "deals the coup de grâce to the everyman theory of consciousness." Nearly everyone, when they introspect their own thoughts, senses that they are "looking inward on an inner space." However, Jaynes submits, there is no such space. There is only physiological tissue. That it is neurological tissue is irrelevant.

You could just as well locate your consciousness in the next room as in your head, Jaynes contends. The localization of consciousness in the brain is arbitrary, because, for example, Aristotle believed that the heart is the abode of consciousness and the brain is merely a cooling organ. To further his case, Jaynes cites the case of a friend who, after regaining consciousness after a left-brain injury, found himself euphorically looking down at his bandage swathed head from a corner of the hospital ceiling. He also cites out-of-body experiences induced by LSD.

Consciousness as Metaphor

"Thus having chiseled away some of the major misconceptions about consciousness, what then have we left?" Jaynes asks the reader. "[D]oes consciousness exist at all?" Jaynes invites the reader to "stare into the dust and rubble" produced by the chiseling to join in the hope that, "Pygmalion-like," consciousness will "step forth pure and pristine out of the detritus." As the "dust settles," Jaynes urges us to "ramble around" and "speak of different things," of metaphors.

Jaynes then rhapsodizes about the wonders of metaphors. They are the "constitutive ground of language." Everywhere we look we find them; in the *head* of an army, table, or bed, in the *face* of a cliff, clock, or crystal, in the *eyes* of needles, storms, or potatoes. They are the engines of enhanced perceptions and understanding. They create new objects.

"Understanding a thing," according to Jaynes, "is arriving at a familiarizing metaphor for it." We designate a familiar object as a *metaphier* and expand its meaning creating a *metaphrand*. For Jaynes, scientific understanding is the "feeling of similarity between complicated data and a familiar model." He cites the Bohr model of the atom in which electrons orbit the nucleus like planets orbiting the sun.

However, the task of finding a metaphor for understanding consciousness confronts a seemingly insurmountable difficulty: "there is not and cannot be anything in our immediate experience that is like immediate experience itself." What is it we are making a metaphor of? We metaphorically speak of a mind-space, with the metaphier being a physical space, "But," Jaynes asks, "if metaphor generates consciousness, rather than simply describes it, what is the metaphrand?"

To navigate this convoluted impasse preventing a metaphorical understanding of consciousness, Jaynes introduces a neologism to describe "various associations or attributes of the metaphier," *paraphiers*. These paraphiers project back into the metaphrand as what Jaynes calls *paraphrands*.

To illustrate this jargon, Jaynes considers the metaphor of snow blanketing the ground. The metaphier is a blanket on a bed. The paraphiers of the metaphier are the associations with warmth, protections, and awakening after slumber. These become the paraphrands of the original metaphrand. Thus, the metaphor of a blanket of snow is enriched, creating the idea of the sleeping earth being protected and warmed until the spring.

The Features of Consciousness

Having explained this layer of complexity underlying metaphors, Jaynes presents his explanation of how metaphors are the stuff of consciousness. Consciousness is both the metaphrand when it is being generated by paraphrands and the metaphier when it acts on unknowns associated with vague memories, present decisions, and future action. This generated structure of consciousness by which we understand the world has the following six features.

First, it is spatialized. When we introspect various images in our "mental space"—trees, birds, or planets—they are spatially separated. Time is also spatialized. If we imagine a timeline of the past hundred years, for example, it typically stretches before our mind's eye from left to right. Second, because we cannot imagine anything in its entirety, we excerpt portions. If we think of a circus, for example, our initial fuzzy image will focus upon a specific feature such as an elephant or a trapeze artist. Our excerptions of people, places, things, and ideas determine our affective responses to them. The third important feature of the structure of consciousness is "the analog 'I'." This is the metaphor we have of ourselves moving about in our imagination doing things that we are not actually doing. The fourth feature of consciousness is the "metaphor me." Not only can the analog "I" look out from within to imagine possible narratives, but it can see itself, the metaphor me, performing specific actions. Narratization is the fifth feature of consciousness whereby various facts, interpretations, and opinions are selected to create a story. Each analog "I" creates its own narrative of the metaphor me on its journey through life. A thief, for example, might narratize his behavior on the basis of poverty and injustice. Gradually we form a coherent image of ourselves that forms the basis for future decisions. We also narratize the actions of others. We see a child, alone, crying in the street and narratize a story of frantic parents searching for him. "Or," as Jaynes notes, "the facts of mind as we understand them into a theory of consciousness." The sixth feature of consciousness described by Jaynes is conciliation. Just as narratization excerpts various elements to create a story enacted in "mind-time," conciliation excerpts them to create conscious objects in "mind-space." Narratization creates stories. Conciliation creates conscious objects by fusing compatible elements of a narrative. For example, an imagined narrative involving a mountain meadow and a tower will conciliate the two objects as a tower rising from the meadow. A mountain meadow and an ocean, in contrast, will not be conciliated but instead be brought together in a narrative involving a succession of events. The conceptual roots of conciliation are behavioral processes whereby an ambiguous perceived object is assimilated into a previously learned schema.

The Mind of Iliad

Having concluded, "Consciousness is this invention of an analog world on the basis of language," Jaynes proceeds to explore its origins. Deeming language to be a uniquely human phenomenon, Jaynes turns his attention to a critical discontinuity in the evolution of language—writing. The central task of his investigation into the origin of consciousness becomes a search for evidence of a subjective conscious mind in the first writings of man.

Translating these hieroglyphic, hieratic, and cuneiform writings from 3000 BC is problematic. We risk projecting our own subjective consciousness into the ambiguities of the marks on stone, clay, or papyrus. According to Jaynes, the first texts that can be translated with sufficient clarity to allow us to search for evidence of subjective consciousness is the *Iliad*, an epic poem which developed from an oral tradition of bards and was written during the eighth century BC. Based on his analysis of its language, he concludes that words such as *psyche*, *thumos*, *phrenes*, and *nous*, which are typically translated as features of subjective consciousness, actually refer to perceptions of physical realities. *Psyche*, for example, does not refer to soul or the conscious mind, but to blood or breath. From the prevalence of commanding gods in the *Iliad*, Jaynes concludes that the warriors depicted in the *Iliad* were "noble automatons" who were directed by auditory hallucinations.

The mentality of the *Iliad* man lacked subjectivity. He had no awareness of his awareness of the world, no internal mind-space to introspect upon. He lacked true volition or planning. An executive part of his mind called a god commanded a passive follower part called a man. Neither was conscious. Such is the basis of the "bicameral mind." Nonconscious organisms behaving like white blood cells obeying the laws of chemotaxis inhabited the great civilizations of Egypt, India, China, and Mesopotamia. Command auditory hallucination played the role of chemical stimuli.

To help the reader gain a feeling of familiarity for this "preposterous" notion, Jaynes compares unconscious bicameral mentality to driving, reflexively responding to changing traffic conditions. Should a sudden change occur, such as a flat tire, we would consciously plan a course of action. Our bicameral ancestors, however, would have had to have waited for "the stored-up admonitory wisdom of his life," to unconsciously tell him what to do.

However, unlike the silent unconscious guidance of the modern driver, Jaynes suggests that the gods who commanded our bicameral ancestors spoke to them. He compares these voices of the gods to the command auditory hallucinations of schizophrenics or the surprisingly prevalent auditory hallucinations heard by normal individuals. Above a certain threshold of stress, the voices of the gods were released. These voices compelled our obedience, because unlike voices of other people we could not escape them. Furthermore, bicameral cultures placed these voices at the top of the hierarchy of political power.

The Bicameral Mind

Recognizing that a completely different kind of mentality organized around unconsciously perceived command auditory hallucinations, existing only a hundred generations ago, "*demands* some explanation of what is going on physiologically," Jaynes explores the neuropsychology of speech. First, Jaynes ponders the mystery of the localization of speech in the posterior third of the left upper temporal lobe, Wernicke's area. Based on the positing of civilizations organized around the bicameral mind, Jaynes concludes that language evolved in the left hemisphere to leave the right side "free for the language of the gods." The right upper temporal lobe communicated with the left via the anterior commissure, a tract of nerve fibers that travels across the amygdala and hypothalamus to the left temporal lobe. Here, Jaynes contends, "is the tiny bridge across which came the directions which built our civilizations and founded the world's religions, where gods spoke to men and were obeyed because they were human volitions."

Next, Jaynes raises the question of how the function of the neural substrate of the bicameral mind that had organized ancient civilizations for thousands of years could have changed over a short period. The answer lies in the plasticity, redundancies, and multiple controls over various psychological capacities that modern neuroscientific research has revealed. An astonishing case cited by Jaynes to illustrate the psyche's ability to recruit neural circuits for its own purposes involved an individual with a congenital absence of the hippocampal fimbria, fornix, septum pellucidum, and massa intermedia of the thalamus who had an easygoing personality and led his class in school. It should not be surprising, therefore, that a thousand years of cultural discouragement of bicamerality should cause its neural substrate to subserve a new function — subjective, creative, introspectable consciousness.

Before explaining the origin of consciousness from the breakdown of the bicameral mind, Jaynes explores the origin of the bicameral mind. Starting with the premise that communication is crucial for animals that depend on social cohesion for survival, Jaynes looks at signaling by primates. He argues that our human ancestors relied on primitive vocalizations, such as grunts, barks, and screeches, and facial expressions for about two million years. Then, as they migrated from the African savannah into the Eurasian subarctic, selective pressure promoted the development of language.

First, about 100,000 years ago, *Homo sapiens* developed intentional auditory signaling. By varying the intensity of a call, varying a cry from "whaee" to "wahoo", for example, one could signal whether a tiger was near or far. Later, about 40,000 years ago, they developed commands and modifiers, as evidenced by archeological remains of sharpened tools. Nouns developed between 25,000 and 15.000 BC as evidenced by cave paintings, pottery, and ornaments.

Each new stage in the development of words created new perceptions and attentions, which resulted in cultural changes. This era coincided with a rapid enlargement of the frontal lobes.

Auditory hallucinations, Jaynes believes, "were a side effect of language comprehension which evolved by natural selection as a method of behavioral control." With the advent of agriculture came the first towns. No longer did groups consist of about twenty hunters and gatherers living in the mouths of caves, but several hundred people living in communities. They built homes with plastered stone walls, paved floors, and reed roofs.

The First Bicameral God

When chiefs could no longer govern effectively with face-to-face encounters, a new method of governance developed. As direct communication with the chief diminished, his hallucinatory voice became his surrogate. These auditory hallucinations, while strictly tied to the ruler's commands, soon began to improvise, thereby allowing for greater behavioral flexibility. Auditory hallucinations were crucial for social order. Suppose, writes Jaynes, that a man is commanded by his chief to set up a fish weir upstream. Lacking consciousness, the man will forget his task. Therefore, he will need auditory hallucinations to remind him what to do.

Stress among the mourners following the king's death intensified his hallucinatory presence. His corpse continued to emanate hallucinatory commands. His burial site became a shrine. This "hallucinogenic king" became humankind's first god.

Jaynes supports this conjecture with evidence from recent excavations of an 11,000-year-old town north of the Sea of Galilee in Israel. There, in the center of a 16-foot diameter tomb, lay two skeletons presumed to be the king and his wife. They are propped up with stones. The tomb was surrounded by a red-ochered structure and covered with large flat stones upon which a hearth was built. Circular stone structures surrounding the hearth were later added. Thus, the paradigm of worshipping gods and constructing pyramids, ziggurats, and temples was established. The problem of succession, as generations of kings were buried, was solved by replacing corpses with statues. These idols became hallucinatory control centers governing unconscious subjects.

Having presented his theory that societies governed by bicameral minds are possible, Jaynes turns to the "witness of history" to support his contention that "such a mentality did in fact exist wherever and whenever civilization first began." Jaynes gathers archeological evidence from various ancient civilizations, from Jericho, to Ur, to Catalhüyük, and Teothihuacan, to support his belief that the magnificent central structures around which towns were organized housed idols or dead kings whose hallucinatory voices commanded nonconscious automatons. Ancient texts refer to the dead as gods. They were buried with food and drink, weapons and tools. From the appearance of figurines, such as large eyes, rituals involving washing out the mouths of idols, and texts which refer to individuals hearing idols speak, Jaynes finds evidence that idols took over the role of broadcasting the voices of the gods.

Writing, according to Jaynes, did not merely visually represent words. The stone engravings of words actually spoke their meanings. The original eight-foot high black basalt stele on which the Code of Hammurabi was written, for example, spoke its edicts. Furthermore, Hammurabi did not compose the eponymous code. It was dictated to the pre-conscious leader by the god Marduk.

While writing as an emitter of hallucinatory commands helped sustain the bicameral system of governance, it also sowed the seeds that contributed to its demise. While the auditory commands of the bicameral mind were wired into the neural circuitry of the perceiver and therefore unavoidable, the voices emanating from words chiseled in stone could be avoided by moving away from them.

The Causes of Consciousness

For thousands of years, the hallucinatory voices of the gods ruled nonconscious automatons organized in a stable hierarchy reinforced by rituals, untouched by outside disturbances. Then during the second millennium BC, the bicameral order began to collapse. As societies grew, the hierarchical network that transmitted the commands of the gods became too complex to manage. It collapsed like a house of cards.

Jaynes envisions encounters between peaceful cultures as promoting harmony. The gods, happily overseeing the smooth tilling, planting, harvesting, and storage of crops would speak beautiful words of peace and harmony. Tentative exchanges of friendly gestures between individuals from different cultures would eventually lead to the exchange of gifts. Thus, trade began.

However, the gods could not cope with forced encounters with unstable cultures resulting from migrations triggered by natural disasters such as droughts or volcanoes. The gods, limited in their range of response to threatening environments, issued commands to kill and conquer. Chaos, bloodshed, and conquest ensued.

Amidst this chaos, protoconscious man unconsciously sensed something within the newly encountered strangers was responsible for their contrary behaviors. From this unconscious inference of an inner consciousness in others, he inferred his own inner world of conscious experience. During these encounters with other civilizations, the gods learned to narratize past experience. Thus, the right temporal lobe became the unconscious repository of what would become conscious narratization by the left temporal lobe. Deceit, the ability to behave one way while internally plotting a secret course of action, is the origin of the analog "I". Instead of automatically following the god's commands to strike out at a man raping one's wife and thereby risk being killed, for example, our protoconscious ancestor would feign acquiescence and survive another day to plot his revenge.

Natural selection played a small role in the origin of consciousness from the breakdown of the bicameral mind. Consciousness, according to Jaynes, is learned behavior. Each new generation must learn how to be conscious. Thus Jaynes claimed, "if you took any child today, and could give me an island and 200 actors and let me construct a culture with an expectation of hearing voices the way I have described it, I could bring up a modern child to be bicameral." The small effect of natural selection was a Baldwin effect; those who were genetically more susceptible to learning consciousness were more likely to survive during the breakdown of the bicameral mind.

Jaynes finds the first evidence of the breakdown of the bicameral mind, the loss of the hallucinatory voices of the gods, in a carving from 1230 BC. A stone altar made by the Assyrian king Tukulti-Ninurta I depicts something dramatically different from anything that had preceded it in the history of the world, a king kneeling, groveling before an empty throne. This represents the loss of the immediate direct communication with the gods during the bicameral era. Confronted with lost divinities, our ancestors searched for ways to make contact with them. Religion was born.

Prayer was unnecessary in the bicameral era. The commanding, hallucinatory voices of the gods immediately filled the space between a desire, a need, or an intention and the act. After the voices fell silent, our ancestors began to pray. Angels and demons filled the vacuum left by the departed gods. Visual depictions of angels, often hybridized with animals, replaced the silenced voices. When the silence of the gods was interpreted as anger, evil demons first appeared in human history. The gods themselves, formerly dwelling in shrines, ziggurats, and pyramids, now ascended skyward to a new heaven.

During the emergence of consciousness—the creation of an introspectable mind-space wherein an analog "I" could use metaphors to narratize alternative courses of action—our bicameral ancestors developed methods of reconnecting with the lost gods. They saw omens in the sequence of natural events. Texts with warnings such as, "If a man unwittingly treads on a lizard and kills it, he will prevail over his adversary," proliferated endlessly. Sortition, which sought to ascertain the divine will by casting lots, and augury which saw god's will in the patterns of oil in a bowl, smoke, or the shapes and colors of organs from sacrificed animals were other methods of divination used during the breakdown of the bicameral mind.

Because, in Jaynes's view, language created consciousness, evidence of the transilience from bicameral unconsciousness to subjective consciousness comes from the earliest writings. Ambiguities and uncertainties regarding the meanings of Egyptian hieroglyphics carved on 5,000-year-old bones and ivory or similarly ancient Sumerian cuneiform tablets, however, are currently unreliable witnessing of early human mentality. Nevertheless, Jaynes finds evidence of proto-consciousness in the letters of Babylonian kings, the spatialization of time in the writings of the first historians, and in the subjective dialogues in the epic of *Gilgamesh*.

The Intellectual Consciousness of Greece

For Jaynes, the clearest, albeit incomplete, literary record of the creation of consciousness by language comes from ancient Greece. Amidst the perplexing, chaotic collapse of the Mycenaean Greek civilization between 1200 and 1000 BC, ancient Greeks created epic poetry to narrate the breakdown of the bicameral mind and the origin of consciousness. "Poems," as Jaynes poetically describes them, "are rafts clutched at by men drowning in inadequate minds." This unique factor is responsible for the fluorescence of Greek consciousness that continues to illuminate the intellectual consciousness of humankind.

According to Jaynes, various words in Greek poetry, such as *thumos, phrenes, nous,* and *psyche* evolved from descriptions of objective physical phenomena to descriptions of subjective consciousness. As bicamerality broke down, as the gap between the voices of the gods and action increased, the ancient Greeks became increasingly aware of the physiological responses to stress, pounding heart, sweaty palms, and rapid breath. These were "pre-conscious hypostases," that would evolve into words referring to conscious planning and intention. They evolved in a succession of four phases:

First, these pre-conscious hypostases referred to external observations; second, they refer to internal sensations; third, the bodily sensations are referred to metaphorically as internal spaces; and fourth, the preceding hypostases are synthesized into a conscious self. The most commonly used word in the *Iliad, thumos,* for example, first describes a warrior who simply sees that a spear piercing his foe causes his actions to cease. Next, as Achilles encounters a novel threatening situation, he becomes more aware of his internal sensations associated with the release of adrenalin, the fight-or-flight response. Then, his *thumos* is metaphorically described as a "container" for one's strength and is implicitly referred to in personal terms. Finally these various hypostases coalesce into the analog "I".

The *Odyssey*, which follows the *Iliad*, reflects a radical leap of mentality. Whereas the characters of the *Iliad* were stimulus-bound, responding automatically to physical stimuli, the characters of the *Odyssey* deliberated over their actions. The frequency of mind-like words, *nous* and *psyche*, increases dramatically and acquire characteristics of consciousness. Odysseus becomes a wily character.

The culmination of the progression of language from descriptions of stimulus-bound objectivity to reflective, deliberative subjectivity is the "invention of the soul." *Psyche*, which refers to life in the *Iliad*, evolves to mean a consciousness that survives death in the *Odyssey*. This change of the meaning of *psyche* from a life force to a disembodied consciousness created a tension in its relationship to *soma*, which had referred to a corpse. *Soma* came to mean body and *psyche* came to mean soul. Thus, as the pre-conscious hypostasis *psyche* began generating metaphors that became the operators of consciousness, the duality between mind and matter, what Jaynes calls "one of the great spurious quandaries of modern psychology," was born.

The Moral Consciousness of the Khabiru

Having examined Mesopotamian relics and Greek poetry for evidence of the transition from pre-conscious bicamerality to subjective consciousness, Jaynes turns to the writings of the ancient Hebrews, the Old Testament. It is, according to Jaynes, an account of the transition from bicamerality to consciousness from the ninth century up to the beginning of the fifth century BC, a story of the chaotic disintegration of the authoritative voices of hallucinatory gods.

Toward the end of the second millemium BC, throughout the Middle East, "large amorphous masses of half-nomadic peoples" roamed the desert wilderness. Most were refugees from the Thera destruction, the Dorian and Assyrian invasions, and the fall of the Hittite civilization. Violent clashes of civilizations had shattered the hierarchical order organized around the bicameral mind leaving these desperate refugees in search of a new order. Joining these refugees were resistant bicameral individuals who could not silence the hallucinatory gods. Shunned, sometimes even killed, by their fellow city dwellers, who were now following the rules of the new consciously governed societies, these remnants of the shattering bicameral era were forced into the wilderness.

These desperate, wretched outcasts sometimes banded together into unstable tribes who raided, fought, or offered themselves as slaves. Some clung to the edges of settled lands to breed sheep and camels. While others "pushed out into the open desert where only the ruthless survive, perhaps in precarious pursuit of some hallucinated vision, some back parts of a god, some new city, or promised land." Cuneiform tablets written in the Akkadian language of Babylon referred to these desert outcasts as *khabiru*, or vagrants: "And *khabiru* softened in the desert air becomes *hebrew*."

The "story or imagined story of the later Khabiru or Hebrews is told in what has come down to us as the Old Testament." It is the story of the loss of the bicameral mind and its replacement by subjective consciousness over the last millennium BC. While Jaynes exults that, when we interpret the Old Testament from this point of view, "the entire succession of works becomes majestically and wonderfully the birth pangs of our subjective consciousness," he also is also concerned about an "orthological problem of immense proportions." Karl Pearson introduced the term orthology in 1882 in *The Grammar of Science* to refer to the "right use of language" so that it would transcend normative meaning and bridge the gap between science and art. For Jaynes, the orthological problem presented by the Old Testament is that it is "well known that much of the Old Testament, especially the first books, are forgeries of the seventh, sixth and fifth centuries BC, brilliant workings of brightly colored strands gathered from a scatter of places and periods." To support this assertion, Jaynes points to the two different creation stories told in Genesis, the similarity between the Sumerian and Biblical story of the flood, and an anachronism involving the stories of Jacob and Joseph.

According to Jaynes, the stories that have come to us in the Old Testament originated in 621 BC with King Josiah's discovery of the manuscript of Deuteronomy during the repairs to the First Temple in Jerusalem. Josiah's religious reforms were a cleansing of the remaining bicameral rites. "Khabiru history," writes Jaynes, "like a nomad staggering into a huge inheritance, put on these rich clothes, some not its own, and belted it all together with some imaginative ancestry." Thus, Jaynes wonders if the Old Testament can serve as evidence of any theory of the mind.

Amos and Ecclesiastes

To assuage skeptics, Jaynes proposes that there are some "pure" books of the Bible that are not compilations. "[T]o these a thoroughly accurate date can be attached." Amos, dating from the eighth century BC, is the oldest such pure book. Ecclesiastes, from the second century BC, is the most recent. The former is an example of "almost pure bicameral speech." Amos is never introspective. When he speaks of himself, he is factual and abrupt. He tells us that that he did not aspire to be a prophet. He was a "gatherer of sycamore fruit," before the Lord called him to prophecy. He does not ponder his prophecies but forcefully speaks the unequivocal words of the Lord.

Ecclesiastes reflects an opposite mentality: "He ponders things as deep in the paraphrands of his hypostatic heart as is possible." He, unlike Amos who relies on divine revelation, speaks of the vanities and vicissitudes of life from his own contemplations. Ecclesiastes surveys the follies and vanities of life using creative metaphors. His poetic teaching, "To everything there is a season, and a time to every purpose under heaven," reflects that spatialization of time that is characteristic of consciousness. Amos and Ecclesiastes represent the extremes of the mentality depicted in the Old Testament that Jaynes believes reflect breakdown of the bicameral mind and the origin of consciousness.

Elohim, the Fall, and the Prophets

Having thus overcome the orthological problems arising from using the Old Testament as evidence for a theory of the origin of consciousness, Jaynes goes on to make several pertinent observations. First, Jaynes asserts that the ancient Hebrews were polytheists. *Elohim*, the word used to refer to God as the creator of heaven and earth in the opening of Genesis, is mistranslated as God. It should be translated as "the great ones, the prominent ones, the majesties, the judges, the mighty ones, etc." From the perspective of Jaynes's theory, the creation story of Genesis is a "rationalization of the bicameral voices at the edge of subjectivity." "In the beginning God created the heavens and the earth," becomes, "In the beginning the voices created heaven and earth."

As the Pentateuch was being stitched together, the large number of hallucinatory gods decreased. Yahweh, translated as "He-who-is," became the most important god. "Evidently," Jaynes concludes, "one particular group of the Khabiru, as the subjective age was approaching, was following only He-who-is, and rewrote the elohim creation story in a much warmer and more human way, making He-who-is the only real *elohah*."

The story of the Fall is a myth of the breakdown of the bicameral mind and the origin of consciousness. The Hebrew word *arum*, used to describe the serpent who tempts Eve to eat from the forbidden fruit from the Tree of Knowledge, means crafty or deceitful. Deceit is a hallmark of subjective consciousness. And after Adam and Eve had eaten on the Tree of Knowledge "eyes of them both were opened," which refers to the opening of "their analog eyes in their metaphored mind-space."

The translation of *nabiim* as prophets is misleading because it connotes telling the future. The true significance of the Biblical prophets is that they overflowed with the visions and words communicated to them by God. They were transitional men who could employ either a bicameral or a subjective mentality. However, the deliverance of God's divine visions and messages was involuntary. God spoke through the prophets. His word was like a fire in one's heart, a fire shut up in one's bones that cannot be contained (Jeremiah 20:9).

The End of Prophecy

Having placed Yahweh, the Fall, and the prophets in the context of the breakdown of the bicameral mind, Jaynes next tells the story of the prophets' vanishing from history. First, as the bicameral mind broke down, there was a loss of the visual component. The earliest Biblical descriptions of God walking in the Garden, shutting the door of Noah's Ark, and wrestling with Jacob are, in Jaynes's telling, visual hallucinations.

By the time of Moses, the visual component of God's hallucinatory presence receded. With the exception of God speaking to Moses "face to face, as man speaketh to his friend" (Exodus 33:11), He now appears as a burning bush, a cloud, or a pillar of fire. The bicameral voice rationalizes the loss of seeing God by saying to Moses, "No man shall see me and live." As the bicameral experience of God recedes further, as His hallucinatory presence becomes accessible only to few semi-bicameral men, the greatest teaching of the Old Testament was revealed: God becomes "something written upon tablets, he becomes law, something unchanging, approachable by all, king and shepherd, universal and transcendent."

As the hierarchical order of the nomadic Hebrews continued to disintegrate, the hallucinatory gods no longer cooperated. It became increasingly difficult to determine which voice had final authority. Moses asserted the authority of his hallucinated voice by producing "magical proofs of his mission" such as "hallucinat[ing] his rod into a serpent or his healthy hand into a leprous one and back (Exodus 4:1–7)." Our current fascination with magic, Jaynes speculates, might derive from the thrill of recognizing the magician as a possible bicameral authority.

After magical signs were no longer available to the prophets to provide evidence of the authenticity of the divine messages they heard, the situation became more problematic. Jaynes cites the example of the "somewhat ridiculous competition between Hananiah and Jeremiah as to whose bicameral voice if the right one."

Not only were the bicameral voices becoming inconsistent between persons, but they were inconsistent within persons. To support this claim, Jaynes cites God's reply to Moses's plea to see His glory: "I will be gracious to whom I will be gracious, and will show mercy on whom I will show mercy." This reply, writes Jaynes, reveals a "bicameral voice [who] is often as petty and foot stompingly petulant as any human tyrant under questioning." God's preference for Abel over Cain, his slaying of Er, and his command to Abraham to sacrifice his son Isaac resemble the impulses by which "criminal psychotics might be directed today."

Further evidence of the breakdown of the bicameral mind is divination. As the authority of voices began to break down, the ancient Hebrews turned to casting *gorals* or lots to divine God's will. This practice involved tossing sticks, bones, or stones with specific markings and interpreting the outcomes as revelations of God's will. The origins of this practice, according to Jaynes, lie with earlier "spontaneous divination from immediate sensory experience." As uncertainty began to take hold in the bicameral voices, they, like men, needed visual inputs to prime their decision-making processes. For example, when Jeremiah sees a boiling wind-blown pot facing north, the hallucinatory god receives this visual input from the right cerebral hemisphere and speaks metaphorically about an evil invasion coming from the north (Jeremiah 1:13–15). When he sees two baskets of figs, one good and one bad, the hallucinatory god inside his head metamorphoses about choosing between good and bad people (Jeremiah 24:1–10).

According to Jaynes, the Book of I Samuel, which dates to the eleventh century BC, was written in the sixth and describes the psychology of the eighth during which time the full spectrum of transitional mentalities was on display. "Wild gangs of nabiim," "winnowed chaff of the Khabiru" were roaming the hills following voices inside their heads they believed to be divine prophecies, stoking their frenzies with drums and music. The book of Samuel tells of Samuel's anointing of Saul as the first King of Israel and King David's succession in the context of the fading of prophecy. In Jaynes's telling, Samuel was a partly bicameral boy trained in the bicameral mode by the old priest Eli. Saul was a "gaunt bewildered country boy whisked into politics at the irrational behest of Samuel's bicameral voice," who struggles to feel the presence of the Lord and follow Samuel's prophecies. David, further removed from bicamerality, practices deception, a hallmark of subjectivity. His first wife, Michal, took a household idol and a covering of goat hair, and placed it in her husband's bed to deceive Saul's agents. The presence of such an idol "may point to some common hallucinogenic practice." After a frenzied, groveling, despairing quest to follow dead Samuel's words, facing military defeat by the Philistines, and conflicts with David, Saul falls on his sword. David becomes King of Israel.

Further vestiges of the disintegrating bicamerality are various "hallucinogenic statuary that are mentioned throughout the Old Testament." Most important are the *tselem*, statues often made from melted gold or silver. Other hallucinogenic idols included *pesels*, carved statues such as the *atsob* worshipped by the Philistines, and *teraphims*, such as the small figurines stolen by Rachel from her father Jacob.

Bicamerality persisted until the era of the fall the Judean monarchy, the Babylonian exile, and the construction of the Second Temple in Jerusalem. The Old Testament was not only the story of the birth pangs of consciousness but the death throes of bicamerality. The story has been suppressed by the authors of the Old Testament who allegedly stitched the story together in the sixth or fifth century BC and, therefore, the fate of the last of the bicameral communities is largely unknown. However, they pop up in the Old Testament as "glimpses of a strange other world."

According to Jaynes, these strange, wild, decadent creatures are often referred to as "son of nabiim," implying a genetic basis for persistent bicamerality. This genetic predisposition for command auditory hallucinations, Jaynes suspects, has persisted as part of the etiology of schizophrenia.

To illustrate the wretchedness of the remaining communities of *nabiim*, Jayne cites I Kings 22:6 which tells how Ahab, "the king of Israel summoned the prophets, about 400 of them, and asked them, 'Should I go to war against Ramoth-gilead, or should I hold back?'" and I Kings 22:10 which tells how, "Dressed in their royal robes, the king of Israel and Jahoshaphat, king of Judah, were sitting on their thrones at the threshing floor by the entrance of the gate of Samaria, with all the prophets prophesying before them." In Jaynes's paraphrasing, the first incident becomes "Ahab, king of Israel in 835 BC, rounded up 400 of them like cattle to listen to their hue and clamor", and the second becomes, "Later, in all his robes, he and the king of Judah sit on thrones outside the gates of Samaria and have hundreds of these poor bicameral men herded up to them, raving and copying each other even as schizophrenics in a back ward."

Sometimes, according to Jaynes, the last remnants of bicameral communities "were hunted down and exterminated like wild animals." For example, I Kings 18:4 describes how Obadiah hid 100 *nabiim* in caves to save them from Jezebel's killing of the prophets. Later, Elijah kills the prophets of Baal (I Kings 18:40).

Eventually, only individual *nabiim* remained. They were partly subjective, yet could still hear the bicameral voice. These individuals include Amos, the exemplar of bicamerality portrayed in the "pure" Book of Amos, Jeremiah, who prophesized the fall of Jerusalem as a consequence of turning away from the Lord, and Ezekiel, who described heavenly visions.

Finally, by 400 BC bicameral prophecy is nearly extinguished. The subjective thought of moral teachers such as Ecclesiastes and Ezra replaced it. The final elimination of bicamerality was achieved by threats of violence: "And if anyone still prophesies, then his father and mother who gave birth to him will say to him, 'You shall not live, for you have spoken falsely in the name of the LORD'; and his father and mother who gave birth to him will pierce him through when he prophesies" (Zechariah 13:3). Such injunctions, if carried out, would "move the gene pool toward subjectivity." By 432 BC, Malachi, the final prophet, died.

Thus, the Old Testament becomes the story of the breakdown of the bicameral mind and the origin of consciousness. The remaining bicameral gods, the *Elohim*, retreat into silence. Confusion and violence ensue. The vain search for the lost gods finally ends.

Reviewing his analysis of the Old Testament, Jaynes concludes that it is our fullest and longest account of the "birth pangs of our subjective consciousness." Chinese literature, which traces its origins into the mists of prehistory, leaps to subjectivity in the writings of Confucius, 551–479 BC. Similarly, the prehistoric oral traditions of the "bicameral Vedas" jumps to the "ultra subjective Upanishads," 800–200 BC. Greek literature, like a "series of steppingstones from the Iliad to the Odyssey and across the broken fragments of Sappho and Solon toward Plato is the next best record, but is still too incomplete."

Jaynes concludes his interpretation of the Old Testament with a passage from Psalms 42:

> As the stag pants after the waterbrooks,
> So pants my mind after you, O gods!
> My mind thirsts for gods! for living gods!
> When shall I come face to face with gods?

This psalm, he says, is evidence that we still are "haunted" by the unconscious longing for "lost authorities." The "deep hollowing yearning for divine volition is with us still."

Vestiges of the Bicameral Mind in the Modern World

Ultimately, prophecy and idolatry were buried under the debris of the collapsed bicameral order. However, its haunting legacy, an unconscious longing for our lost bicamerality, the source of religion, remained. Having provided textual and archeological evidence of a bygone era when our pre-conscious ancestors were ruled by command auditory hallucinations produced by the right temporal lobe, Jaynes examines its vestiges. In the immediate aftermath of the breakdown of the bicameral mind, oracles channeled the lost gods. "Oracles were subjectivity's umbilical cord reaching back into the sustaining unsubjective past," perhaps represented by the conelike structure called the *omphalos*, or navel, located at the reputed center of the earth at the Temple of Apollo at Delphi. Here the gods spoke through the high priestesses. Their channeled responses to questions posed by kings ruled the world.

To explain this astonishing phenomenon, Jaynes introduces "the general bicameral paradigm." It consists of four aspects. First is the *collective cognitive imperative*, a culturally constructed set of beliefs, expectations, and procedures that define the significance of rituals such as the divination of the Oracle of Delphi. Second is an *induction*, a ritualized procedure that narrows consciousness toward a specific goal, and third is the resulting *trance* which diminishes the analog "I" so that it can fulfill its culturally defined role. Fourth is the *archaic authorization*, the connection of a god to a powerful leader who empowers the oracle to rule. For nearly a millennium, tens of thousands of pilgrims from the Mediterranean world came to the awesome cliffs of Delphi to feel the numinous presence of divine energies surge through them.

As bicamerality faded and skepticism grew, the collective cognitive imperative that sustained oracular power crumbled. New ways of reconnecting heaven and earth such as Gnosticism and Neo-Platonism developed. However, attempted revivals of old ways, especially idolatry, filled the gaps that new beliefs could not fill. Whereas previously, idols spoke to nonconscious bicameral worshippers, they now spoke to subjectively conscious, rational individuals. This bizarre practice was sustained by the now universal belief in the dualism of body and spirit. If a disembodied divinely created soul could animate a material body, it could also speak through idols.

Another phenomenon that developed in the aftermath of the breakdown of the bicameral mind was possession. While bicameral prophets relayed their hallucinatory voices to their listeners, speakers in the throes of possession experience their utterances as coming directly from their vocal apparatus. They are completely dominated by the gods who speak through them and do not allow recollection of their words. Unlike the nonconscious bicameral speaker who first hears his word as auditory hallucinations, the possessed speaker enters a new realm of consciousness wherein his words are articulated externally.

Related to possession is glossolalia. Here a rhythmic pressured stream of purportedly divinely inspired words spoken in a language unknown even to the speaker erupts from an unknown source. These utterances resemble the rhymes of epic Greek poetry and provide a window into the true language of the gods.

Jaynes rhapsodizes that the gods were the first poets. The Muses were not imagined, they were experienced. Even today, poets experience their verses as erupting from the wellsprings of creativity beyond conscious control. Consciousness, imitating the gods, jealously suppresses inspirations from lost gods. They vanish in the instant one consciously tries to apprehend them. The "grinding tides of irreversible naturalism have swept the Muses even further out into the night of the right hemisphere," until we doubt their inspiration.

Related to possession, insofar as it involves a diminution of the sense of self and the overtaking of the ego by forces beyond it, is hypnosis. Because hypnosis show that consciousness can be radically altered by the seemingly "ridiculous ministrations" of a hypnotist, Jaynes argues that consciousness cannot be the immutable product of neural processes that evolved hundreds of millions of years ago. Rather, it is a learned, malleable phenomenon. Hypnosis allows us to tap into the lost authority of the bicameral mind.

Schizophrenia, with its auditory hallucinations, dissolution of ego boundaries, and the diminished capacity for narrative thinking, is, according to Jaynes, a relapse to the bicameral mind. However, while our bicameral ancestors were nonconscious components operating an integrated hierarchical theocracy, schizophrenics experience the terror and panic of witnessing the implosion of their conscious selves. There was no setting apart of others as mentally ill because back in the bicameral era everyone was schizophrenic. Initially, as described in Plato's *Phaedrus*, the persistence of hallucinatory control of mentality was viewed as a "divine gift." But later, in times of war and famine, when consciousness originated from the breakdown of the bicameral mind, hallucinating individuals were pathologized and shunned. Schizophrenics struggle to adapt to the conscious constructs of modern culture. They are "waiting on gods in a godless world."

Neurologically, schizophrenics share the cerebral laterality of the bicameral mind. The right hemisphere dominates both the schizophrenic and bicameral brain. This proposed vestige of the bicameral mind can be investigated with modern neuroimaging devices.

The Auguries of Science

Jaynes concludes his discussion of the vestiges of the bicameral mind by asserting that science is a nostalgic quest for the lost authoritative directives of the bicameral mind. Science and religion, therefore, share a common source. The conflict between science and religion derives from dispute between the methods of the Church and those of empirical science. The Church relies on vanished revelation codified in ancient traditions and texts. Science relies on deductive and inductive reasoning and the verification and falsification of theories based on observation.

Until the nineteenth century, most scientists believed that they were exploring God's intellect as it is revealed in Nature. Then, in what Jaynes calls the Great Human Irony, "our noblest and greatest endeavor on this planet" led to the discovery that "in our reading of God in Nature, we should read there so clearly that we have been wrong all along." Beginning with the French Enlightenment and culminating in a manifesto led by the German physiologist Hermann von Helmholtz, materialism expelled spiritual entities, vital forces, and divine substances from scientific discourse.

The rise of Darwinism greatly accelerated this profaning of the holy. Blind chance and natural selection operating on matter, not divine intelligence, were the creators of man. We are alone in a godless world.

The dissolution of the ecclesiastical authority led disillusioned individuals to seek new sources of meaning beyond themselves. Scientology, astrology, meditation, and psychedelics filled the void. In addition to these attempts to replace lost authority of the clergy, the "Great Human Irony" is that humankind's travels along the road of science, "our noblest and greatest endeavor on this planet," ends with the realization that we have been actually searching for the lost authority of the hallucinatory voices that commanded our nonconscious ancestors. In an ironic twist on science's ironic embrace of materialism along the road believed to have been leading to God, science transformed into quasi-religious scientisms such as materialism, psychoanalysis, and behaviorism. These scientisms acquired the trapping of religion; all encompassing explanations, charismatic leaders, dogmatic canonical texts, and the marginalization of "heretics."

Karl Marx's studies of class struggles in France under Napoleon led to dialectic materialism and communism, which usurped religion's power. It promised atonement for man's fall from paradise with a return to a lost "social childhood of mankind where mankind unfolds in complete beauty." Psychoanalysis took cases of the relief of symptoms of hysteria by analyzing repressed sexual memories and elevated their role to a "central superstition" that could explain civilization and its discontents. The God of Abraham, Isaac, and Jacob was explained as the unconscious projection of one's father, the feared, awe inspiring main character in a repressed sexually charged childhood drama.

Each of these scientisms contains a kernel of truth. But they overreached to explain everything and thereby became superstitions. The "nostalgia for the Final Answer, the One Truth, the Single Cause," seduces followers into religious fervor. We are fervently and vainly searching for a spurious lost innocence.

No individual is "so abject a creature as to have any conscious articulate willing to reach either the absolutes of gods or to return to a preconscious innocence," Jaynes proclaims. Instead we are at the mercies of inescapable cultural forces generated by the silent hallucinatory voice of the gods. "The very notion of truth," he declares, "is a culturally given direction," "an outgrowth of the search for lost gods in the first two millennia after the decline of the bicameral mind."

Summary

In summary, Jaynes proposes that no forms of life—from the 3.7 billion year-old cyanobacteria to the poets who composed the Iliad—were conscious. Auditory hallucinations supplemented other nonconscious adaptive mechanisms in humans about 14,000 years ago. Voices spoken by Wernicke's area in the right temporal lobe, perceived as gods, commanded our nonconscious ancestors. This "bicameral mind" broke down about 1,000 years ago because of clashes between civilizations and natural disasters. Metaphorical language, the stuff of consciousness, rose from the shattered ruins of the bicameral mind. Vestiges of our lost bicamerality remain. Schizophrenics are commanded by voices in their heads. Religion and science nostalgic searches for lost hallucinatory gods.

Two

Origins of The Origins of Consciousness in the Breakdown of the Bicameral Mind

Julian's father, Reverend Julian Clifford Jaynes, cautioned that, "The man who thinks he knows it all, excludes the light with the wall of his own conceit." He "simply closes the door to truth, and the great world passes on and leaves him in a self-made tomb." Seeking to heed his father's warning against the sin of pride, Jaynes concludes his flamboyant tale of the origin of consciousness by acknowledging that his essay is not immune to the unconscious lure of the lost hallucinatory gods. However, this apparent humility derives from the conceit that those gods are "real."

In my opinion, Jaynes's theory is what Carl Wernicke, whose eponymous area is the dominant counterpart of the conjectured source of the hallucinatory gods of the bicameral mind, termed an "overvalued idea." Such ideas are cathected with intense intellectual and emotional energy and are dissociated from conflicting evidence and logical inconsistencies. Neurologically, overvalued ideas operate within "closed circuits" with loosened associations with other areas of the brain. Wernicke coined the term sejunction for this loosening of association fibers. Psychologically, overvalued ideas are preoccupying for the individual but are neither obsessions nor delusions. Philosophically, overvalued ideas straddle the infamous boundary separating pseudoscience from science that continues to perplex those trying to solve the demarcation problem.

While the comparison of Jaynes's theory to an overvalued idea has pathologizing connotations, it also connotes the possibility of genius. Jaynes's theory continues to resonate with a deep chord in the human psyche—our longing to understand our innermost selves, the origins and nature of human consciousness, and the origins of religion and science. However, ultimately it fails to explain the origins of consciousness. By better understanding the origins of the *The Origin of Consciousness in the Breakdown of the Bicameral Mind*, we might open new neural circuits and shine new light into the self-made tomb of the bicameral mind.

Jaynes's father died when he was two. Whether owing to the repression of infantile sexually charged dramas, poverty of language, or rapid hippocampal neurogenesis, Jaynes, like all infants, had no conscious memories of his father. The "spiritual presence" of his father began to take shape when he would delve into the 48 volumes of his father's sermons. Nearly every sermon ended with a prayer to our "Heavenly Father." The first metaphor for God that Jaynes encountered had no feelings of familiarity for him. Jaynes would become an atheist for whom God was an hallucinatory voice.

But Reverend Jaynes's sermons not only had the unintended effect of leading his son toward atheism. They inspired him to challenge the "very suspicious totem of evolutionary mythology" that human psychology has evolved continuously from worms to apes to man. He told his congregation:

> To feel that he is merely a clay image marooned on a planetary cinder, flings him back to the ape or tiger. To look up at white stars in the darkened heavens, to read the message of his own heart yearnings and to discover in both nothing more than omnipotent *matter* rolling on relentlessly to sure doom, pitiless and dark, is not a philosophy that exalts the soul or saves it from the lust of selfish power.

And, not only did Reverend Jaynes inspire his son to search for the spark that ignited humankind's launch along a trajectory at right angles to Darwinian evolution, but he pointed to the time of the launch. In a sermon extolling the spiritual powers of the soul that can lift individuals above the vicissitudes of fate, beyond heredity and environment, Reverend Jaynes wrote:

> We sometimes speak of environment and heredity as if they were the equivalent of the old Greek Destiny that even pulled the strings which actuated the hands of the Olympian gods, but there is no destiny except what a man creates for himself. A man's fate does not reside on Olympus, where Zeus hands down to him weal or woe, light or darkness.

This metaphor of environment and heredity acting as if they were the equivalent of old Greek Destiny, that even pulled the strings which actuated Zeus who metes out man's fate, took a peculiar twist in young

Julian's mind. The Greek gods became auditory hallucinations commanding nonconscious ancient Greeks.

The idea that the people described in the first written record of Greek gods and warriors were literally nonconscious puppets had its roots in Jaynes's early career as a behaviorist. While Jaynes abandoned behaviorism because "Nobody really believed he was not conscious," he convinced himself that the Greeks before 1000 BC were not conscious.

While Jaynes dismisses his involvement with behaviorism as a misguided first attempt to understand consciousness, his colleague and co-author, Stevan Harnad, referred to an "earlier besottedness with behaviorism." The lingering effects of that "besottedness" led him to eliminate all elements of consciousness until only metaphorical language, the only tangible reflection of his father's spiritual presence, remained.

Jaynes's early besottedness with behaviorism not only caused him to chisel away all elements of consciousness except metaphorical language but also created "closed circuits" and "disjunctions" that distorted his perceptions. For example, he incorrectly paraphrased of John Locke's aphorism, "Nothing is in the intellect that was not first in the senses," as "There is nothing in consciousness that is not an analog of something that was in behavior first." Jaynes's assertion that "concepts are simply classes of behaviorally equivalent things" reflects an overvaluation of behaviorism that bewilderingly pushes concepts into the realm of the nonconsciousness. However, entangling himself in what Douglas Hofstadter famously referred to as a "strange loop," Jaynes responds to criticism that he is confusing the concept of consciousness with consciousness itself by replying that he is fusing them because they are the same. The most bewildering lingering effect of his early besottedness with behaviorism is his assertion that "we can only know in the nervous system what we first know in behavior."

Jaynes's "besottedness" with behaviorism began as a student when he fell under the spell of what he would later recall as a "kind of huge historical neurosis," associationism. According to Jaynes, this doctrine, which developed during the eighteenth and nineteenth centuries, identified consciousness with an actual space wherein sensations and ideas associate. This association constitutes learning, which is equated with consciousness and experience. Thus to study the evolution of consciousness is to study the evolution of learning.

Convinced, at the time, that the study of the evolution of learning is indeed the study of the evolution of consciousness, Jaynes began his scientific career trying to condition a mimosa plant to droop its leaves in response to an intense light. Jaynes concluded that the "long-suffering" plant was "not conscious." Next, he tried to condition individual paramecia to navigate a T-maze engraved in wax on black Bakelite by punishing its errant turns with electrical shocks. Following this failure to demonstrate consciousness in paramecia, Jaynes moved on to species with synaptic nervous systems, such as worms, fish, and reptiles. After several years, he concluded that this effort to chronicle the evolution of consciousness by studying conditioned learning was "ridiculous." Consciousness is what we introspect. And when we introspect, it is not upon conditioned responses. Why, he wondered, did so many distinguished scientists pursue this ridiculous path toward understanding consciousness, and why was he "so lame of mind as to follow them?" The answer, he concluded, was that the theories had been so attractively presented by such prestigious champions that they became embedded in culture.

Eager to cast off the chains of his youthful indoctrination, Jaynes embraced behaviorism. Unlike associationism, which sought an explanation of consciousness, behaviorism excluded consciousness from the halls of science. Jaynes introduces the reader to behaviorism's "startling doctrine" that consciousness doesn't exist by tracing its rise to dominance to the toppling of idealism following World War I, the longing for objectivity comparable to physics, and the effete opposition offered by it nearest rival, Titchenarian introspectionism. Eager to sweep aside the obfuscating theories of the past, psychologists turned to the clear objectivity of conditioned responses and operant behaviors.

During the time of Jaynes's scientific training, behaviorism dominated academia, "and set its arrogant banners up in one university after another." Those who attempted to address the problem of consciousness were banished from academic psychology and texts hid the problem from view. But, as Jaynes notes and as was mentioned earlier, "Nobody really believed he was not conscious." Behaviorism was a method, not a theory. While Jaynes rejects behaviorism as a perverse denial of consciousness, he does believe that it successfully swept away the muddled theories of the past. Psychology could tackle the problem of consciousness with a fresh start.

Eager to make such a fresh start, Jaynes first tackles the problem of determining what consciousness is. Under the influence of his behaviorist indoctrination, he chisels away all the self-evident elements of consciousness, including consciousness of consciousness, perception, thinking, and reasoning, until only a web of metaphiers, metaphrands, paraphrieires, and paraphrands remained.

Having thus defined consciousness, Jaynes searches for its origin. Again, under the influence of behaviorism, he asserts that consciousness originated from nonconscious puppets whose strings were pulled by the Greek gods. Having started at one end of the spectrum where plants and paramecia are conscious, he leaps to the other where only humans living after 1000 BC are conscious.

And, if metaphors are the stuff of consciousness and the ancient Greek authors of the Iliad were nonconscious poets writing about nonconscious puppets, then the gods could not be metaphors for fate, destiny, and free will. Who, then, were the gods?

The answer came to Jaynes in his late twenties, living alone in his Boston apartment "autistically pondering" the problem of consciousness, "circling about the sometimes precious fogs of epistemologies, finding nowhere to land." A "distinct loud voice from his upper right" provided his epiphany. This auditory hallucination told him, "Include the knower in the known."

Thus, under the partially suppressed influence of behaviorism and an epiphanous auditory hallucination, the metaphorical Greek puppets of Reverend Jaynes's sermons, ruled by the Olympian gods, became, for Jaynes, actual nonconscious puppets commanded by auditory hallucinations. This psychological model then found its neural home in the newly discovered dual brain. The currently nonverbal right brain was once the source of command auditory hallucinations. It fed those commands from Wernicke's area across the anterior commissure.

Jaynes rhetorically asks, "Apart from this theory, why are there gods Why religion? Why does all ancient literature seem to be about gods, and usually heard gods?" He does not consider the possibility that there is a God and His prophets communed with Him. While Reverend Jaynes urged his congregants to find inspiration to climb that "great altar stair that slopes through the darkness up to God ... the Eternal, Infinite, Absolute Good of whose sprit every human spirit is born," his son believed that this stairway to heaven leads to the illusory paradise of lost hallucinatory gods. Jaynes's search for God follows the closed circuits that generated the theory of the bicameral mind. It travels within the walls of his self-made tomb constructed from the conceits of his certitude about the bicameral mind. However, while Jaynes excluded light within the walls of his own conceit and closed the door to truth, leaving himself in a self-made tomb, the light generated by his genius, the light he shined on that recent explosion of consciousness when the first dialog between man and God began, can illuminate new pathways connecting the knower, knowledge, and the object known.

The Great Human Irony, according to Jaynes, is that man's search for God along the road of science led to materialism and atheism. In a subsequent ironic twist, the spiritual void created by the death of God was filled by inflating various scientisms such as psychoanalysis, behaviorism, and Marxism to quasi-religious proportions. Ironically, Jaynes's efforts to liberate science from its self-deluded quest for illusory divinities and lost innocence entombed him with false certitudes.

Three

Assessment

The Consciousness of Consciousness

To arrive at his astonishing conclusion that consciousness originated 3,000 years ago, Jaynes first tries to persuade us that what we "feel" to be the "most self-evident thing imaginable," that consciousness of consciousness is "the defining attribute of all our waking states, our moods and affections, our memories, our thoughts, attentions and volitions," is wrong. Our beliefs that consciousness is the basis of concepts, learning, reasoning, thinking, and judging are "costumes that consciousness has been masquerading in for centuries," preventing us from finding a solution to problem of the origin of consciousness.

Jaynes begins by "chiseling away" what he regards as misconceptions about consciousness and then proposes that, "Pygmalion-like," a new conception of consciousness rises from the detritus. First, he chisels away perception.

Contemplating his assertion that perception is nonconscious reactivity rather than conscious awareness, we are pulled through the looking glass with Alice to confront Humpty Dumpty's theory of words and meaning:

> "I don't know what you mean by 'glory'," Alice said.
> Humpty Dumpty smiled contemptuously. "Of course you don't—till I tell you. I meant 'there's a nice knock-down argument for you!'"
> "But 'glory' doesn't mean 'a nice knock-down argument'," Alice objected.
> "When *I* use a word," Humpty Dumpty said, in rather a scornful tone, "it means just what I choose it to mean—neither more nor less."
> "The question is," said Alice, "whether you *can* make words mean so many different things."
> "The question is," said Humpty Dumpty, "which is to be master—that's all."

Jaynes recounts how, at a meeting of the Society for Philosophy and Psychology, "a well-known and prestigious philosopher" vociferously objected to his contention by exclaiming, "I am perceiving you at this moment. Are you trying to say that I am not conscious of you at this moment?" But Jaynes dismisses his response, concluding that he was only conscious of the rhetorical argument he was making and would have been better conscious of him if he had turned his back or closed his eyes. According to Jaynes, a "collective cognitive imperative in him" was answering in the affirmative. The question is, as Humpty Dumpty correctly pointed out, which is to be the master of meaning. But, to assert that perception is nonconscious reactivity is tantamount to asserting, Humpty-Dumpty-like, that "glory is a nice knock-down argument." The "collective cognitive imperative," the dictionary meaning of words, is the basis of meaningful communication.

Jaynes's justification for rejecting the dictionary definition of perception is his assertion that perception is solely the behavioral response to an environmental stimulus. To use Jaynes's example, should a bird noisily burst up from a nearby copse and distract him from his writing, he might turn and watch it and hear it, and then return to his writing. All this would occur, according to Jaynes, without his conscious awareness. However, while unconscious reflexive behavior might initially draw his gaze toward his window, his subsequent focus on the bird's flight, appreciation of its natural beauty, assessment of its classification, are all elements of conscious perception. The return to his writing and search for his train of thought entails conscious volition.

Consciousness differentiates perception from mere physical reactivity. The hard problem of consciousness is why, for example, the pathway from photochemical reactions in the retina, to neural spikes along the optic nerve, to the network of electrochemical activity in the occipital cortex, participates in the consciousness of visual sensations while the pathway from the lens of a video recorder to the storage of electronically coded pixels, for example, does not. More importantly, Jaynes's central thesis that consciousness arose from command hallucinations broadcast to nonconscious individuals relies on the same denial. "Hallucinations" broadcast to nonconscious individuals, he asserts, are merely neural spikes, not voices. However, the idea of nonconscious hallucinators is oxymoronic.

Concepts, Learning, Thinking, and Reasoning

Jaynes argues that there is no necessary connection between concepts and consciousness. Jaynes arrives at this conclusion by redefining concepts: "Concepts are simply classes of behaviorally equivalent things." Such equivalent behaviors—bees seeking nectar, for example—are the result of genetically programmed instincts. Jaynes proposes to replace the term instinct, which is generally used to refer to fixed patterns of behavior in response to specific stimuli, with the term "aptic," which he defines as "organizations of the brain ... that make the organism apt to behave in a certain way under certain conditions." However, just as perception is not mere reactivity, concepts are not simply classes of behaviorally equivalent things. Concepts are generalizations or abstractions of experiences often unrelated to behaviors. They are the elements of conscious thought.

According to Jaynes, when we consciously think of a tree, we are conscious of a particular tree that grew beside our house, "no one has been *conscious* of *a* tree." However, to consciously think about woody perennial plants is to be conscious of a tree.

While Pavlovian conditioning can influence our affective and motor responses, such behaviors are a small subset of learning. Teaching differential equations by Pavlovian conditioning would not likely promote learning.

While the participants in Marbe's experiments were not conscious of the neural events along the proprioceptive and tactile pathways leading to conscious sensations, or even the deliberations regarding the relative weights of the objects, they were conscious of those sensations and they consciously evaluated them according to their understanding of the instructions. Sudden flashes of insight experienced by mathematicians and scientists sometimes erupt from the depths of the unconscious. But those unconscious eruptions were fueled by prior conscious rumination and become meaningful only when they rise to the level of conscious awareness. It was not until Einstein had consciously pondered expanding his theory of special relativity based on inertial reference frames to accelerating reference frames for several years that his "happiest thought," the equivalence of gravity and acceleration, burst from his unconscious. This insight was developed into the general theory of relativity only after years of arduous thinking and calculations.

Jaynes's examples merely show that unconscious processes participate in mental activities. While excessive self-consciousness can be a hindrance to the performance of learned behaviors such as playing the piano, consciousness sets the goal, evaluates our successes and failures, and monitors and adjusts the optimal level of self-awareness.

Self-Blind Chiselings

Jaynes's assertion that "Consciousness is a much smaller part of our mental life than we are conscious of, because we cannot be conscious of what we are not conscious of" is false. One's consciousness of the percentage of one's mental life that is conscious varies according to the lens through which one sees consciousness. A psychoanalyst might see consciousness as the tip of a vast unconscious iceberg. Eliminativists deny that consciousness exists at all. Jaynes exempts himself from the supposed inability to be conscious of the part of our mental life that supposedly eludes our consciousness. We *can* be conscious of what we are not conscious of. Contents from the unconscious reach consciousness along the royal road of dreams, by sudden flashes of intuition, and the recollection of repressed memories. We can voluntarily shift our consciousness from immediate phenomenal awareness. The consciousness of what we are not conscious of is the basis of all our explorations of the unknown.

Jaynes's analogy of consciousness searching its mental life with a flashlight searching a dark room, looking for something that does not have any light shining upon it, breaks down. The flashlight would not conclude that there is light everywhere. The flashlight would see the shadowy boundary between light and dark. It would also "see" the darkness. Indeed, one would not know that consciousness is only part of one's mental activity if one could not turn one's consciousness to an awareness of what one is not usually conscious of.

Consciousness not only includes an awareness of what one is not conscious of, but consciousness of consciousness, and the consciousness of the consciousness of consciousness, and so on, expands consciousness in an infinitely recurring self-referential loop. That consciousness can also be conscious of what one is not conscious of adds another "strange loop" of consciousness.

However, while there would not seem to be any limits towards extending this self-referential loop infinitely, our visual and auditory representations begin to flicker and fade by the third iteration. Perhaps the riddle of consciousness can be solved by opening the doors of perception to higher dimensions. Or, perhaps the answer to the riddle of consciousness is beyond the limits of the human mind. Such is the position of the "Mysterians."

We are similarly confronted with the limits of reason in mathematics, which, notwithstanding Jaynes's arguments, requires consciousness. Kurt Gödel, who showed that consistent axiomatic systems of sufficient complexity to contain arithmetic are necessarily incomplete, observed that, "Either mathematics is greater than the human mind, or the mind is greater than a machine."

He believed the latter. Rather than base mathematics on a finite set of axioms, Gödel proposed that that by avoiding the "mistake of letting everyday reality condition possibility and only imagining combinations and permutations of physical objects, the mind is capable of directly perceiving infinite sets," and thereby accomplishing the "goal of all philosophy, the perception of the Absolute." To achieve this perception of the Absolute, "First, one must close off the senses, and actively seek with the mind."

And who is the perceiving, cognizing subject of consciousness? Who is conscious of his own consciousness? Jaynes misconstrues Descartes' "I think, therefore I am" to mean that we are the continuous stream of thoughts that flow before our mind's eyes. It is, in Jaynes's words, "our deepest of deep identity." Because this continuity of consciousness is illusory, as shown by the mind's filling in the gap in the visual field produced by the retinal blind spot, and the perception of a continuous of time in spite of the flickering of neural spikes between neural refractory periods, our deepest identity is an illusion.

However, Descartes did not identify the "I" with the contents of one's consciousness. Indeed, he started with the ultimate skeptical argument that all our perceptions and thoughts could be unreal. The only thing we can know with certainty, by virtue of the fact that we are thinkers, is that we exist. Furthermore, we also know the flickerings of neural spikes as conscious experience. Which is the illusion? Is it the continuity of phenomenal awareness? Or is it the flickering of neurons? Also, given the gaps in our knowledge, one cannot say with certainty that flickering neurons are the physical basis of visual experience.

Jaynes writes that he thinks that the contentless analog "I" is related to Kant's transcendental ego: "As the bodily I can move about in its environment looking at this or that, so the analog 'I' learns to 'move about' in mind space, 'attending to' or concentrating on one thing or another." While there is indeed a relationship between the analog "I" and the transcendental ego, they are not identical. When the analog "I" sees itself as the "analog me," it transcends its status as an analog and spins away from itself in an infinitely recurring self-referential loop as the transcendental ego.

Ludwig Wittgenstein, like Kant, similarly argued, "The philosophical 'I' is not the human being, not the human body, or the human soul of which psychology treats, but the metaphysical subject, the border—not a part—of the world." While Wittgenstein declared that "*The limits of my language* means the limits of my world," and advised "What one cannot speak about, one must pass over in silence," he also declared, "There is of course the unspeakable. It shows itself; it is the Mystical," and "anyone who understands me eventually recognizes [my elucidations] as nonsense, when he has used them—as steps—to climb up beyond them. (He must, so to speak, throw away the ladder after he has climbed it.)"

Illustrating Wittgenstein's warning that "Philosophy is a battle against the bewitchment of our intelligence by means of our language,"

Jaynes writes, "And the feeling of a great interrupted stream of rich inner experiences, now slowly gliding through dreamy moods, now tumbling in excited torrents down gorges of precipitous insight, or surging evenly through our nobler days, is what it is on this page, a metaphor for how subjective consciousness seems to subjective consciousness." Here, again, Jaynes fails to make the distinction between the contents of consciousness, "subjective consciousness," and the subject of consciousness, the transcendental ego, the philosophical "I."

Free Will

Jaynes justifiably rejects the "helpless spectator" theory, according to which consciousness is a mere epiphenomenon of neural activity with no causal potency. Free will lies at the heart of our notion of sanity and moral responsibility. A legally insane individual is one who can neither discern right from wrong nor adhere to the right. The denier of free will who proudly claims to have climbed above the illusion of free will by climbing the ladder of reason refutes his own denial.

However, Jaynes does not take his belief in free will to its logical and empirical conclusions. For Jaynes free will involves creating new arrangements of metaphors from an ever-expanding lexicon. He does not fully explore the role of the brain in these free creations of the mind. While it is inconceivable that consciousness has nothing to do, conceiving how free will controls the brain leads to the conclusion that human consciousness approaches the powers of the God of theism.

Erwin Schrödinger, in his contemplations of free will, grappled with what he believed to be two indisputable premises: 1) "our bodies function as pure mechanisms according to the Laws of Nature." 2) "I know by controvertible evidence that I am directing its motions." He concluded that the only possible inference is "I am God Almighty."

Schrödinger asserts that this declaration sounds "both blasphemous and lunatic" in Christian terminology and is a stranger to Western ideology. However, as he points out, the insight is not new. Mystics, for centuries, independently, have described experiencing a unity with God "in terms that can be" condensed in the phrase: "DEUS FACTUS SUM, I have become God."

Is Consciousness in Our Head?

Jaynes argues that the "everyman theory" that consciousness is in our heads is wrong because it derives from the misguided feeling that when we introspect we are looking inward toward a space behind our eyes. Also, we assume that a similar space exists in others, a "space behind our companions eyes into which we are talking." But, Jaynes warns, "if we press ourselves too strongly to characterize this space (apart from its imagined contents) we feel a vague irritation, as if there were something that did not want to be known, some quality which to question was somehow ungrateful, like rudeness in a friendly place." This feeling, Jaynes proposes, leads us to the conclusion that "we know perfectly well that there is no such space inside anyone's head at all." There is nothing inside our heads except "physiological tissue." "And the fact that it is predominantly neurological tissue is irrelevant."

This discomfiting realization, Jaynes continues, leads us to continually invent spaces in our own heads or other arbitrarily chosen seats of consciousness. Aristotle, for example, located consciousness just above heart and believed the brain to be a mere cooling organ. While the idea that consciousness is in our heads is so deeply ingrained that it is difficult to imagine otherwise, "you could, as you remain where you are, just as well locate your consciousness around the corner in the next room, against the wall near the floor, and do your thinking there as well as in your head." To support this contention Jaynes cites examples of out-of-body experiences.

However, Jaynes's rejection of the localization of consciousness to the brain is refuted by empirical evidence. A "brainectomy" would remove all signs of consciousness. A pinpoint lesion of the reticular activating system can cause coma. Lesion of Wernicke's and Broca's area of the brain can eliminate the capacity for metaphorical speech, the stuff of Jaynesian consciousness. Voluntary actions correlate with physical events in the premotor cortex, not "around the corner in the next room." That Aristotle and others mistakenly located consciousness in the heart is irrelevant. Heart transplants and heart lung machines have disproved this ancient mistake. Saturating the atmosphere of a room around the corner with a potent psychoactive substance has no affect on consciousness. A few micrograms of a potent psychoactive substance flowing through the cerebral vasculature alters our reality.

Jaynes's citing of out-of-body perceptual experiences as a refutation of the idea consciousness is in our head is inconsistent with his assertion that perception does not involve consciousness. His claim that consciousness is metaphorical language is inconsistent with his claim that consciousness is not in our head. Damage to Wernicke's or Broca's areas produces aphasias.

Nonetheless, the anecdotal evidence from out-of-body experiences presented by Jaynes to support the idea that consciousness is not in our heads does raises legitimate questions regarding the possibility that one's perceptions can extend beyond the brain's ordinary sensory inputs. However, while, for example, some near-death experiencers have described their resuscitations from a bird's eye view, the possibility of subliminal sensory inputs has not been conclusively ruled out. Reports of visits to heaven, clearly, might be hallucinations. Even if consciousness can rise from a nearly dead brain to perceive oneself and one's surroundings, or even ascend to heaven, there is a necessary connection to the neural circuits of memory. Séances, channeling reincarnations, and poltergeists notwithstanding, there is no evidence of completely disembodied consciousness. That consciousness is on our heads remains our only current working hypothesis.

For Jaynes, out-of-body experiences "do not demonstrate anything metaphysical whatever; simply that locating consciousness is arbitrary." However, the demonstration of disembodied consciousness would have profound metaphysical implications. A consciousness that has left its customary position of looking out through the eyes to gaze at oneself from the ceiling would challenge the materialist foundations of neuroscience. The location of consciousness in the instance of such veridical out-of-body perceptions would not be arbitrary; it would be localized to a specific location near the ceiling. The numerous reports of near-death experiencers encountering the spirits of the deceased, including those who were not previously known to the individual, or encountering other-worldly realms present further challenges to our metaphysical assumptions.

While the "everyman's theory" that consciousness is in our heads oversimplifies the relationship between mind and matter, Jaynes's dismissal of the localization of consciousness to the brain as an arbitrary, invalid inference based on vague intuitions is unwarranted. Perhaps consciousness is "located" in hyperspatial branes contained in a multiverse. Nevertheless, neural events occurring within the space-time coordinates circumscribed by the brain and the duration between our embryonic development and death irrefutably intersect uniquely with consciousness.

Did Nonconscious Poets Write the *Iliad*?

Homer's lack of "mental language" in the *Iliad* and his prevalent use of objective descriptions of behavior do not justify the conclusion that the characters of the *Iliad* lacked consciousness. While it is true that objective descriptions prevail in the *Iliad*, this prevalence is unsurprising and there are exceptions. Jaynes acknowledges that language almost certainly evolved from nouns referring to direct sensory impressions. The development of language toward the expression of subjective experiences, desires, intentions, and conflicts evolved slowly.

Willard Quine provides the useful metaphor of language as a web whose periphery consists of words that are most closely linked to the triggerings of our sensory neurons. Language began from the periphery of the web, with objective descriptions of external reality. As language evolved, words moved further and further from the triggerings of sensory neurons toward the abstract realms of subjective experience, desires, intentions, and conflicts. According to literary historian Joan DeJean, for example, portrayals of characters underwent a revolution, especially in France, during the late 1600s. Characters were no longer driven by passions seen as external forces acting on passive subjects, but by inner emotions and thoughts. It is not surprising, therefore, that Homer's *Iliad* lacked the rich descriptions of inner life found in Tolstoy or Dostoevsky.

Furthermore, while Jaynes points towards instances where words describing behaviors are focused on objective phenomena, he disregards instances where those words describe subjective phenomena. For example, while Jaynes translates *thumos* as motion or agitation, Hector engages in an internal dialogue with his *thumos*: "Yet still, why does the heart within me debate on these things?" In addition, while Jaynes asserts that deception is a hallmark of consciousness, the supposed nonconscious bicameral originators of the *Iliad* tell us "Athene deceived Hector with her words and her disguise."

Jaynes encounters a similar difficulty when analyzing the *Work and Days* attributed to Homer's near contemporary Hesiod. Jaynes dismisses the scholarly consensus that the poem *Work and Days*—about a farmer railing at his bungling brother Perses for mismanaging the farm he'd inherited from their father, taking him to court, and writing a manual to help salvage the farm—is by Homer. Instead, he proposes that the older portions of the poem dealing with Perses were actually written by the admonishing bicameral voices of Perses himself. "If this jolts your sense of possibility," Jaynes advises you to consider that schizophrenics also hear admonishing voices. However, this interpretation of the authorship of *Work and Days* does little to lessen the jolt to our sense of possibility. That a nonconscious hallucinating Perses wrote, or dictated to a scribe, the words spoken by the voices in his head that were later integrated into a narrative poem written from the narrator's point view strains our credulity to breaking point.

Not only does the idea that the *Iliad* describes automatons obeying auditory hallucinations strain our credulity but it is also contradicted by the text. While the gods are the supreme forces who initiate the actions of the characters in the *Iliad*, there are exceptions that leave the reader to ponder the relationship between fate and free will. While

Achilles is destined to die, he is given the choice of whether to enter the battle, to live a short life with glory or a long life without glory. Similarly, Hector can choose to confront Achilles or flee to the city.

Not only does an analysis of the language of the *Iliad* not support the inference that the characters it describes are not conscious, but also the notion that the *Iliad* was composed from tales transmitted by nonconscious bards defies reason. The bards, like their bicameral contemporaries, were stimulus-bound creatures nonconsciously following neural commands, displaying reflexive adaptation to their environment. How did they know the interior lives of the characters, the voices of the gods that spoke to them? How did nonconscious poets compose a poem that provides a metaphor for the transilience toward consciousness?

Jaynes rejects the argument that the gods are a poetic device to make the action more vivid, replying that it "is the same kind of thing as to say that Joan of Arc told the Inquisition about her voices to make it all vivid to those who were about to condemn her." However, there is a fundamental difference between Joan of Arc speaking about the voices of angels and saints she heard, and Homer writing about the gods that communicated with the heroes of the *Iliad*. Joan of Arc was indisputably conscious. She was speaking from a first-person perspective about her own experiences. Jaynes contends that the bards who sang the epic poems about the heroes of the Trojan War and the poet or poets who composed the *Iliad* had access to the interior lives of others yet were not conscious.

The attribution of Greek theology to auditory hallucinations operating within a nonconscious brain ignores the intellectual history of the origin of the Greek gods as first recorded in Hesiod's *Theogony*. This theogony reflects abstract cosmological speculations, visual imagination, and elaborate dramatic narratives that, by any standard, including Jaynes's, must be attributed to conscious thought. Auditory hallucinations directing stimulus-bound behaviors to nonconscious automatons could not reasonably be said to have composed such a complex, abstract theogony wherein gods acted consciously. The gods cavorted, fought, and schemed within the introspectable mind space of the warriors of the *Iliad*, and therefore those warriors were conscious.

Further weakening Jaynes's argument that Greek gods described in the *Iliad* were command auditory hallucinations is the testimony of the Greek historian Herodotus: "Indeed, wellnigh all the names of the gods came to Hellas from Egypt. For I am assured by inquiry that they have come from foreign parts, and I believe that they came chiefly from Egypt." Regarding the gods themselves, he wrote:

> But whence each of the gods came in to being, or whether they had all for ever existed, and what outward forms they had, the Greeks knew not till (so to say) a very little while ago; for I suppose that the time of Hesiod and Homer was not more than four hundred years before my own; and these are they who taught the Greeks of the descent of the gods, and gave to all their several names, and honors and arts, and declared their outward forms.

This line of transmission of knowledge about the Greek gods starts in the mists of Egyptian prehistory and merges with Hesiod and Homer who gave them names and declared their outward forms. Hesiod and Homer were not describing hallucinations directing nonconscious automatons.

While Jaynes has no problem convincing himself that that the *Iliad* is a tale of nonconscious warriors written by nonconscious poets, he does struggle with believing that the *Odyssey* as a narration of the coming of consciousness was composed, planned, and put together by poets who were not conscious of what they were doing. Countering skeptics, including himself, who "are inclined to ask scoffingly and rhetorically, how could an epic that may itself be a kind of drive toward consciousness be composed by nonconscious men," he claims, "We could also ask with the same rhetorical fervor, how could it have been composed by conscious men?" However, Jaynes's struggle to believe that nonconscious poets wrote about the arrival of consciousness is a struggle with an illusion of his own making. Conscious poets wrote both the *Iliad* and the *Odyssey*. And, even if nonconscious poets wrote the *Iliad*, there would be no reason to fervently ask how an epic about the transilience to consciousness could have been written by conscious men. Who else but a conscious individual could write about the origins of consciousness? Nonconscious poets are mysterious. Conscious poets are not.

While the proposition that hallucinating philosophical zombies battling on the fields of Troy were the mothers of consciousness strains our credulity, a similar theory was proposed by Bruno Snell, holder of a chair for classical philology at the University of Hamburg, in *The Discovery of the Mind: The Greek Origins of European Thought*, published in 1953. The "mind" referred to by Snell is equivalent to Jaynesian consciousness, an introspectable world of thought. Like Jaynes, Snell sees the origin of consciousness in transition from concrete language describing physical sensations and actions to metaphorical language describing the inner world of the mind that began with Homer's poetry. Snell's analysis of the *Iliad's* language led him to conclude: "Homer's conception of *thymos, noos,* and *psyche* still depended to a large extent on an analogy with the physical organs." Also, "Homer does not know personal decisions; even when a hero is shown pondering two alternatives the intervention of the gods plays the key role ... human initiative has no source of its own."

While Snell speaks of the "discovery" of the mind, he uses the term in a way that acknowledges the "strange loop" of consciousness. The Greeks did not discover the mind as "Columbus discovered the New World." Whereas the North American continent had existed long before Columbus discovered it, the mind, Snell concludes, "did not come into existence until it was discovered; it exists by grace of man's cognizance of himself." Nevertheless, Snell justifies this paradox by claiming that the mind is not an invention, which he avers is arbitrarily determined by adapting to goals. However, while Snell claims that no aims were involved in origination of the intellect, clearly the intellect served the goal of navigating our ancestor's way through the unpredictable, frightening chaos of raw sensory experience. Even if we grant Snell the contention that the intellect was not invented, we still, as Snell warns, "encounter two terminological difficulties."

The first is the philosophical problem arising from the claim that the Greeks discovered the mind while also claiming that this discovery was necessary for bringing the mind into existence. Suffice it to say, Snell does not cut through this perennial Gordian knot of self-referential paradoxes. Following a discussion of divine revelation, self-revelation, and discovery, Snell concludes that they are, for all practical purposes, equivalent. They do, however, differ in their historical contexts. Snell prefers discovery to revelation because humankind had to discover the means of communicating what it had apprehended and struggled to preserve. The intellect was born of suffering. Protection from further suffering is a bar to further wisdom.

The second terminological difficulty is analogous to the first, but framed as a philological rather than a philosophical problem. Although the intellect did not come into being until it was "discovered," Snell asserts, "we realize that Homer conceived the thing which we call intellect in a different manner, and that in a sense, the intellect existed also for him, though not *qua* intellect." That "thing" is, unsurprisingly, elusive. Owing to the limits of the translatability of languages, we cannot clearly apprehend the thoughts expressed in alien tongues. Nevertheless, Snell believes that we might "establish contact with Greek thought, not only through the medium of historical recollection, but we may recognize in it the threads of our involved patterns of thinking."

Snell's scholarly tome highlights a remarkable era in the intellectual history of humankind, the flowering of the arts, philosophy, and medicine in ancient Greece. However, the proposition that the Greeks discovered the mind, like Jaynes's theory of the origin of consciousness from the breakdown of the bicameral mind, self-destructs in the whirlpool of strange loops.

Did Advanced Bicameral Civilizations Exist?

Further straining our credulity beyond the notion of nonconscious poets who nonconsciously foretold the coming of consciousness is Jaynes's contention that nonconscious individuals commanded by auditory hallucinations built the Mesopotamian ziggurats, the Egyptian pyramids, and the Mycenaean temples. Originally, tribal leaders ruled their subjects directly by face-to-face interactions. As the expansion of villages made this type of leadership impossible, auditory hallucination evolved to supplement the leader's commands, to encourage perseverance in his absence. These hallucinatory commands were initially like recordings of the leader's voice, but later they improvised. The stress from the leader's death intensified the hallucinations of the bereaved subjects. They erected tombs and believed that the dead leader was the divine source of the hallucinatory voices that commanded them. Later idols replaced the tombs. Which, according to Jaynes, became "the carefully tended centers of social control, with auditory hallucinations instead of pheromones."

The problem with this theory is that, just as the queen bee does not control the hive with pheromones, neither the chief nor his inanimate surrogates broadcasted hallucinatory signals. The hallucinatory voices spoken in the bicameral minds are self-generated. How would the voices know what commands to issue to their nonconscious obeyers as they built the pyramids entombing the mummified pharaohs? Did they direct every hammer blow of each and every quarryman? Did they guide the hand on the rod that removed the deceased pharaoh's brain through his nose? Did they align the massive stones of the pyramids with the stars?

Jaynes is led astray by analogizing the hallucinatory control of nonconscious bicameral minds with the social behavior of bees and termites. Jaynes's analogy of a dead king ruling a bicameral society by auditory hallucinations with a queen ruling a termite colony or a beehive with pheromones breaks down because the queen wields no political power. She only lays eggs. She has no knowledge of what needs to be done and no capacity to control the colony. Research conducted by Deborah Gordon and others during past few decades has shown that the collective behavior of ant colonies is a self-organizing phenomenon governed by responses to rates of interactions among individual ants who communicate their levels of hydration and other variables through olfactory communication.

Self-organizing systems such a termite colonies and beehives repeat patterns determined by environmental variables and fixed algorithms. The advance of human culture from the first cave dwellers to the builders of the ziggurats and pyramids requires creative innovation.

Furthermore, according to Jaynes, the bicameral societal hierarchy immediately decided whether an individual was responding to the correct voice. This was achieved by recognition signals, known to everyone, as to which god was speaking. Priests reinforced the edicts issued by those signals. But if an individual could be mistaken as to whether his bicameral voice was the correct one, how could another individual, a priest or someone of lesser rank, be certain that the voice in his head was correctly interpreting the signal of his neighbor. Also, Jaynes's model of societies governed by hallucinatory voices ignores competing external voices. Verbal behavior from the pre-bicameral persisted and developed during the bicameral era. The bicameral voices not only activated the neural circuits that initiated actions, but also activated the circuits that caused those hallucinatory voices to be spoken. Which voice—the spoken voice of the pre-bicameral era, the voice in one's head, or the verbalized voice of another's bicameral voice—was the correct one?

Does Jaynes Explain the Origin of "Jaynesian Consciousness" from the Bicameral Mind?

Jaynes lures the reader into his complex, extravagant tale of the origin of consciousness by promising to answer the perennial riddle of consciousness: why are some physical states conscious while others are not? However, his proposed nonconscious originator of consciousness (besides possessing nearly the full spectrum of the attributes of consciousness) is physically equivalent to its conscious successor. Owing to the brain's plasticity and redundancy, the same neural machinery is both conscious and not conscious. The nonconscious bicameral mind operates within a brain that is neurally equivalent to the conscious brain. This indifference to the problems raised by placing nonconscious mentality and consciousness in neurally equivalent brains is in stark contrast to his recognition that the "completely different kind of mentality" that characterized the recently lost bicameral mind "demands some statement of what is going on physiologically."

Jaynes not only evades the question of why some physical systems are conscious while others are not, but the proposed sociological origin of consciousness from the breakdown of the bicameral mind is as mysterious as the emergence of consciousness from complex physical systems. His explanation that the observation of different patterns of behavior during encounters with people from other nations led to the inference that something inside them was different, perhaps an inner life, can only be stated ironically by Jaynes: "We may first unconsciously (sic) suppose other consciousness and then infer our own."

According to Jaynes, consciousness originated from auditory hallucinations that commanded nonconscious automatons. However, even if we leave aside the oxymoronic nature of nonconscious hallucinators, we are still left with the problem of how the sights and sounds spoken by nonconscious individuals gave rise to consciousness. While all emergent theories of consciousness confront an explanatory abyss, nonconscious matter does not suffer from the self-contradiction that nonconscious poets does.

Karl Marx also proposed that language is the stuff of consciousness. In *The German Ideology*, written in 1846, Marx writes:

> Language is as old as consciousness, language *is* consciousness that exists also for other men, and for that reason alone it really exists for me personally as well; language, like consciousness only exists from the need, the necessity, of intercourse with other men ... Consciousness is, therefore, from the beginning, a social product, and remains so as long as men exist at all.

However, the proposition that language and consciousness emerged from social interactions suffers from the same lack of explanatory power as the theory of the emergence of consciousness from a network of neurons. The origin of language and consciousness from a network of interacting physical organisms is as mysterious as the origin of consciousness from a network of firing neurons.

Jaynes similarly glosses over the explanatory gap separating nonconsciousness from consciousness when discussing the development of what Jaynes variously refers to as "compatibilization," "conciliation," and "consilience"—the conscious unification of various threads of knowledge. Using Piaget's notion of assimilation, the incorporation of similar experiences into pre-existing ideas—such as grouping an unfamiliar canine into the category of dog—Jaynes asserts, "assimilation consciousized is conciliation." The problem with this assertion is that according to Piaget's theory of cognitive development assimilation is consciousized unconscious reflexive behavior that results from the assimilation of similar stimuli. The assertion that assimilation consciousized is conciliation starts with a false premise (assimilation is nonconscious), and does not explain how nonconscious assimilation gives rise to conscious consilience.

According to Jaynes, the dualism between mind and body is a "spurious quandary" that originated from a "tension in the lexicon" of the words used during the progression from the *Iliad* to the *Odyssey*. The word *psyche*, for example, transformed from a life force that simply left the body upon death to a disembodied soul that could enjoy the afterlife and reincarnate other bodies. Jaynes confesses that he is "unable to suggest a truly satisfactory solution" to the problem of how this semantic transformation occurred. His attribution of this notion to Pythagoras avoids the question of how he developed the concept. He rejects Herodotus's proposal that he learned the idea from the Egyptians. This suggestion, Jaynes believes, rests on a misunderstanding of the Egyptian words *ba* and *ka*. Based on the theory of the bicameral mind, *ba* refers to the persistence of the physical embodiment of the hallucinatory voice of *ka*. Here, again, we are confronted with the unsolved problem of how consciousness originated from a noncomscious source.

Jaynes's theory of the origin of consciousness relies on emergentism. However, unlike conventional theories of emergence, which date the emergence of consciousness at 500 million BC, Jaynes dates the threshold of emergence at 1000 BC. This recent dating of the origin of consciousness arouses our misgivings because it seems self-evident that individuals who created advanced civilization were conscious. But even if they were not conscious, Jaynes's contention that metaphors generated consciousness requires an unjustified inversion of reasoning. Metaphors do not generate consciousness. Consciousness generates metaphors.

Metaphors are empty vessels until individual consciousness gives them meaning. For example, while Jaynes interprets the "tinsmith's scoop" in Seamus Heaney's poem "Sunlight" as a metaphor for "the whole simulating (and so paraphranding) sexual intercourse from a male point of view," the poet Melissa Reeser Poulin interprets it differently:

> With the sound of that scoop in our ears, its muted bite into coarse grain, we muse out loud. Yes, love is like that: sunk into the *work* of life. With our hands full of struggle, slowness, pieces and fragments, we make our lives. Over time and with the blessing of years, the making becomes inextricable from our loving, our being loved.

Even more astonishing than the proposition that metaphors create, rather than reflect, consciousness is the idea that metaphors create the transcendental ego. A self-referential web of metaphiers, metaphrands, paraphiers, and paraphrands creates its creator.

Does the Search for the Physical Basis of Consciousness Follow a Delusional Line of Reasoning?

Jaynes's search for the origin of consciousness in the transition of language from auditory hallucinations commanding actions to internal metaphorical dialogs was motivated, in large part, by his conclusion that the search for the physical basis of consciousness follows a "delusional line of reasoning." To arrive at this conclusion, Jaynes starts with the perplexing assertion that, "We can only know in the nervous system what we have known in behavior first." Less perplexingly, but irrelevantly, Jaynes goes on to state that even if we had a complete wiring diagram of the brain, even if we knew the connections of every synapse together with all their neurotransmitters, we could still never —"not *ever*"—from knowledge of the brain alone know if that brain contained a consciousness like our own. But this merely states the obvious. The neuroscientific search for the physical basis of consciousness correlates objective measurements of neural events with subjective reports of internal states. The hope is that as those correlations grow stronger, the explanatory gap between objective, external, physical reality and subjective, internal, mental reality will close. Nevertheless, Jaynes concludes that we must start from the top down, from a clear conception of what consciousness is. Only then can we enter the world of neurology.

After chiseling away what he believes consciousness is not, Jaynes beholds consciousness as an ever-expanding web of mataphiers, metaphrands, paraphriers, and paraphrands. If Jaynes's top-down approach to solving the riddle of why some physical systems are conscious while others are not is to succeed, he must explain why consciousness understood as metaphorical language can enter some physical systems while it cannot enter others. But Jaynes offers no explanation. Consciousness understood as metaphorical language and nonconsciousness understood a command auditory hallucinations are equally at home in the same brain. Culture determines which brain is conscious and which is not.

Both the bottom-up and the top-down approach reach an impasse when we follow what Jaynes rightfully calls the all too common and unspoken tendency to translate psychological phenomena into neuroanatomy and neurochemistry. However, if we dig deeper into the physical activity of the brain we arrive at the quantum mechanical level. Quanta are both the highest mental abstractions and the bedrock of physical reality. "We are suspended in language in such a way," said Niels Bohr, "that we cannot say what is up and what is down."

For nearly one hundred years scientists have pondered the possibility that the search for the most fundamental level of physical reality leads to consciousness. The bottom is the top. While Jaynes does not directly refer to quantum mechanical theories of consciousness, he does allude to them in his rejection of "consciousness as a property of matter." According to Jaynes, physical theories of consciousness attracted mostly physicsts during the "historical epoch" when "[t]he solidity of matter was being dissolved into mere mathematical relationships in space, and this seemed like the same unphysical quality as the relationship between individuals conscious of each other." However, Jaynes dismisses physical theories of consciousness because they answer the wrong question. Physicists explain physical interactions between objects and their environment including measuring devices. They do not explain our introspectable conscious experience.

However, while it may turn out that quantum mechanical theories of consciousness are based on nothing more than a vague affinity between the immateriality of mathematical abstractions and consciousness, the dissolution of solid matter into mathematical relations in hyperspace is a profound mystery that might hold the secrets of consciousness. While Jaynes maintains that the 1913 Bohr model of the atom remains, physicists discarded it during the 1920s. There are no concrete visualizable models that represent the atom. There is no quantum ontology. There is only an epistemology based on mathematics. In spite of quantum mechanics' remarkable success, profound, fundamental questions remain. What are quanta made of? How do they materialize into classical realities? Do quantum effects affect consciousness? Does consciousness affect quantum effects? While it is true that a current wiring diagram of the brain cannot, alone, tell us if that brain "contain[s] a consciousness like our own," it is possible that a quantum mechanical one could.

Quantum Orthodoxy

Quantum orthodoxy, based on the Copenhagen Interpretation formulated by Niels Bohr and Werner Heisenberg, declares that quantum mechanics provides only a mathematical formalism that allows us to predict the probability of the occurrence of an actual reality. The equations tell us nothing about an actual quantum reality. As Bohr famously declared, "There is no quantum world. There is only an abstract quantum description." It is meaningless to discuss what happens inside the atom. We can only discuss the outcomes of measurements of atomic phenomena using classical concepts. "The use of classical concepts is finally a consequence of the general way of thinking. There is no use in discussing what could be done if we were other beings than we are," declared Heisenberg.

When Einstein first encountered quantum orthodoxy, he seems to have been receptive to the idea that a new understanding of the relationship between consciousness and physical reality could create a window into the quantum world. In 1926, during a walk with Heisenberg, the latter defended his position that only observables could be used to describe atomic events. Einstein countered:

> You must appreciate, that observation is a very complicated process. The phenomenon under observation produces certain events in our measuring apparatus. As a result, further processes take place in the apparatus, which eventually and by complicated paths produce sense impressions and help us fix the effects in our consciousness. Along this whole path—from the phenomenon to its fixation in consciousness—we must be able to tell how nature functions, must know the natural laws at least in practical terms, before we can claim to have observed anything at all.

When Heisenberg protested to Einstein that he had based relativity on observable phenomena, he replied one should not repeat the same joke twice. Ironically, one of the inspirations of relativity was Karl Pearson's *The Grammar of Science*. Pearson speculated that an observer traveling at the speed of light of light would perceive the eternal now. An observer traveling faster than light would observe events traveling backward in time. However, for Pearson, unlike for Einstein, these relativistic effects tell more about the human mind than objective reality. "In truth," he wrote, "the field of science is much more about consciousness than an external world."

In his 1936 essay, "Physics and Reality", Einstein, after acknowledging the logical impossibility of differentiating between "sense impressions and images," wrote, "With the discussion of this problem, which affects also the notion of reality, we will not concern ourselves, but we shall take the existence of sense impressions as given, that is to say, psychic experiences of a special kind." These sense impressions can never be guaranteed to be "anything other than an illusion or hallucination." However, they are touchstones of reality for the physicist. Einstein ultimately rejected the idea that we can open the "doors of perception" and perceive the quantum world.

Einstein was instrumental in developing quantum mechanics. His 1905 Nobel Prize winning discovery of the laws of the photoelectric effect led to the acceptance—in the face of opposition by Max Planck and others — of the particle nature of light. He was the first to propose wave/particle duality. His recognition of the significance of Louis de Broglie's theory of matter waves led to its acceptance. Erwin Schrödinger acknowledged the "brief but infinitely far seeing remarks by Einstein," and that his method of deriving his wave equation "means nothing less than taking seriously the de Broglie-Einstein wave theory of moving particles." Max Born, who showed that the Schrödinger equation is a tool for calculating the probabilities of the outcomes of measurements wrote that the "decisive step was taken once again by Einstein ... who showed that the classical concept of intensity of radiation must be replaced by the statistical concept of *transitional probability.*"

However, Einstein famously refused to accept quantum mechanics as the "true Jacob," as a complete description of physical reality, and despaired of finding one. In 1911, Einstein replied to a visitor's question about the wildly gesticulating people who could been seen from his office, "Those are the madmen who do not occupy themselves with the quantum theory." That same year, Einstein wrote to his friend Besso, "I no longer try to construct quanta because I know now that my brain is not capable of it."

Nevertheless, after his successful generalization of relativity converted him to the belief that reality could be grasped with mathematics as the "ancients dreamed," Einstein searched for a mathematical description of microscopic reality that would go beyond the fuzzy ontology of quantum orthodoxy. He accused Bohr of being not only a "mystic," but also a "Talmudic philosopher [who] doesn't give a hoot for 'reality' which he regards as a hobgoblin of the naïve." In a 1928 letter to Erwin Schrödinger, shortly after Bohr's interpretation of quantum mechanics became dogma, Einstein wrote, "The Bohr-Heisenberg tranquilizing philosophy — or religion? — is so delicately contrived that, for the time being, it provides a gentle pillow for the true believer from which he cannot very easily be aroused. So let him lie there. ... Most of them simply do not see the risky game they are playing with reality. ... Hardly any of the fellows can get out of the already accepted concepts, instead, comically, they can only wriggle inside." Twenty-five years of constant brooding about quantum mechanics only intensified his opposition. When he looked up at the moon, he asked his fellow physicist and future biographer Abraham Pais, "Do you really believe the moon is not there when you are not looking?" In 1952 Einstein wrote to his friend and fellow physicist Daniel Lipkin, "This theory reminds me a little of the system of delusions of an exceedingly intelligent paranoiac, concocted of incoherent elements of thought."

Einstein often expressed his vision of scientific truth beyond the limits of quantum theory in religious language. In 1926, he wrote to Max Born, "Quantum mechanics demands serious attention. But an inner voice tells me that this is not the true Jacob. The theory accomplishes a lot, but it does not bring us closer to the secrets of the Old One. In any case, I am convinced that He does not play dice." In 1948, he wrote to his friend Michael Besso, "that in spite of its great practical successes, I do not consider the present statistical quantum theory a good approach. It's the same with me as the Jews with the 'Messiah'." In 1951, he told his assistant Ernst Strauss, "What really interests me is whether God could have created the world any differently; in other words, whether the logical simplicity admits of a margin of freedom."

Einstein-Podolsky-Rosen Paradox

During the 1980s, physicists carried out experiments that actualized a variation of a 1935 thought experiment proposed by Einstein, in collaboration with Boris Podolsky and Nathan Rosen, to show that quantum mechanics is incomplete. When two quanta interact and then fly apart, then, according to quantum mechanics, they become entangled; the measurement of one quantum instantaneously determines the properties of the other. Therefore, quantum mechanics implies that physical reality does not exist independent of its observation, and the transformation of quantum abstractions to physical reality can occur via a "spooky action at a distance." Both of these implications are "unreasonable" and therefore, Einstein argued, quantum mechanics is "incomplete."

By shining lasers into non-linear crystals, physicsts created entangled photons. Measurements of their polarizations were made along various angles. Using a mathematical analysis developed by J.S. Bell — Bell's Inequality — physicists showed that it is impossible to reproduce the predictions of quantum mechanics using a theory of local hidden variables.

Because of Einstein's rejection of "spooky action at a distance " — "non-local interaction" — most physicsts have declared that Einstein was wrong regarding his assessment of quantum mechanics. However, the demonstration that the setting of one measuring device influences the reading of another instrument in a way that cannot be explained by the transmission of local signals does not disprove Einstein's position that quantum mechanics is incomplete. Indeed, nonlocal interactions of entangled quanta are not possible unless they are unreal until they are observed. Which is the basis of Einstein's opinion that quantum mechanics is incomplete.

Because physicists have assumed that adding local hidden variables to the existing conceptual structure of quantum mechanics is the only way to complete it, they believe that we are compelled accept quantum descriptions of reality as complete. But Einstein's arguments were not based on hidden variables:

> It is my opinion that the contemporary quantum theory of certain definitely laid down concepts, which on the whole are taken over from classical physics, constitute an optimum formulation of certain connections. I believe, however, that this theory offers no useful point of departure for future development. I think it is not possible to get rid of the statistical character of the present quantum theory by merely adding something to the latter, without changing the fundamental concepts about the whole structure.

Nathan Rosen, his collaborator, agreed: "If quantum mechanics is replaced by another theory, this is likely to involve revolutionary changes in concepts and principles ... It appears that such a theory won't be obtained from simple modifications, such as hidden variables."

Furthermore, Einstein wanted to replace quantum mechanics' *Subcausalitat* (subcausality) with *Ubercausalitat* (supercausality). Such a theory would replace the "choice" of experimenter with a predetermined "decision." Such "super-determinism," as Bell explained in a 1985 BBC interview, would obviate the need for faster than light signals.

Beyond Quantum Mechanics

While quantum mechanics' fuzzy ontology and problematic epistemology argue against its completeness, it is unclear whether revolutionary new concepts can ever completely grasp reality as it exists independent of its observation. In a letter to Einstein following the *Festschrift* held to celebrate Einstein's seventieth birthday that continued the debate started during the 1927 Solvay Conference when Bohr replied to Einstein's statement that "God does not play dice with universe" by telling him to stop telling God what to do, Bohr wrote:

> To speak in the same jocular tone, I cannot help saying about the disquieting questions, that to my mind the issue is not whether we should cling to a reality which is accessible to physical description, but rather, we should pursue the path shown by you and discover the logical prerequisites for the description of the realities. In my impertinent manner,

> I would even go so far as saying that no one—not even the dear Lord himself—can know what the phrase like playing dice means in this context.

Einstein soon reached a similar conclusion:

> All the fifty years of conscious brooding have brought me no closer to answer the question, "What are light quanta?" Of course today every rascal thinks he knows the answer, but he is deluding himself.

Einstein was not proven wrong about his belief that a more complete description is possible, but he did fail to find one. His search for a unified field theory that would unify our understanding of gravity and electromagnetism deterministically in a way that preserved the idea of physical reality existing independent of its observation eluded the highest flights of Einstein's genius:

> My opinion is that if the objective description through the field as an elementary concept is not possible, then one has to find a possibility to avoid the continuum (together with space and time) altogether. But I have not the slightest idea what kind of elementary concepts could be used in such a theory.

Bohr, from whose vanished model the new quantum theory arose, flirted with the idea of extending quantum mechanics to include consciousness. As recalled by Heisenberg, Bohr once said:

> We can admittedly find nothing in physics or chemistry that has even a remote bearing on consciousness. Yet all of us know there is such a thing as consciousness, simply because we have it ourselves. Hence, consciousness must be part of nature, or more generally, of reality, which means that, quite apart from the laws of physics and chemistry, as laid down in quantum theory, we must also consider laws of quite a different kind. But even here, I do not really know whether we need a greater freedom than we already enjoy thanks to the concept of complementarity.

However, while Bohr did not know whether the concept of complementarity affords the freedom needed to accommodate consciousness within the laws of physics and chemistry as laid down by quantum mechanics, it is clear that if consciousness and physical reality have the same complementary relationship as the waves and particles of quantum mechanics, then they would spin away from each as mutually exclusive realities. Not only would mind and matter spin away from each other, but also, as Bohr first realized during a childhood encounter with the Licentiate of Paul Martin Møller's unfinished novel, *A Danish Student's Tale*, consciousness itself spins away from itself:

> Furthermore, I come to think of my thoughts about it, indeed I think about my thoughts thereof and I devote myself into an eternally descending line of "I's" who observe each other. I do not know at which "I" I must stop and in the moment I stop at one, there is again an "I" which does the stopping. I become confused and feel dizzy as if I looked into a bottomless abyss.

"If you can fathom quantum mechanics without getting dizzy, you don't get it," said Bohr. Similarly, if you can fathom the hard problem of consciousness, why some physical systems are conscious and others are not, without getting dizzy, you don't get it. Bohr also referred to the parallels between the challenges faced by quantum mechanics when confronting our roles as both "spectators and actors in the great drama of existence" and the "psychophysical parallelism envisaged by Leibniz and Spinoza," or "even to that kind of epistemological problems with which already thinkers like Buddha and Lao Tse haven been confronted." However, Bohr went on to distance himself from accepting a role for consciousness. Conflating consciousness and "mysticism," he wrote:

> Still the recognition of an analogy in the purely logical character of the problems which present themselves in so widely separated fields of human interest does in no way imply acceptance in atomic physics of any mysticism foreign to the true spirit of science.

In his last discussion about the relationship between quantum mechanics and consciousness, Bohr wrote:

> Indeed in renouncing logical analysis to an increasing degree and in turn allowing the play on all strings on emotion, poetry, painting and music, [we discover that the latter] contain possibilities of bridging between extreme modes of those characterized as pragmatic and mystic. Conversely, already ancient Indian thinkers understood the logical difficulties in giving exhaustive expression to such wholeness.

Complementarity resigns us to the position that mind and matter cannot be united. Mysticism, understood as a subject experiencing the unity of the knower and the known, no longer confronting an independently existing objective reality, is indeed foreign to the true sprit of science. However, the turn to emotion, poetry, painting, and music does not contain possibilities of bridging pragmatism and mysticism. It only soothes our dizziness when gazing into the abyss.

Curiously, while Bohr rejected "mysticism," Einstein chided him for being one. Referring to Bohr's denial of reality to phenomena described by Schrödinger's equation, Einstein wrote:

> There is also the mystic, who forbids, as being unscientific, an inquiry about something that exists independently of whether or not it is

observed, i.e., the question as to whether or not the cat is alive or at a particular instant before an observation is made. (Bohr)

Here, of course, Einstein is referring to "Schrödinger's cat," whose fate is tied to a quantum system, a radioactive atom that could trigger the release of a vial of cyanide. According to quantum mechanics, the atom exists as a superposition of being decayed and undecayed until the atom is observed. Therefore, the cat is both dead and alive until the atom is observed.

To label Bohr a mystic for forbidding an inquiry into the cat's fate before triggering the radioactive atom is observed as unscientific is puzzling. A mystical experience is a purportedly supersensory perception of realities that are not accessible to ordinary sensory perception and therefore a mystic would not forbid an inquiry into the status of that which is unobserved. Nor, as someone who seeks to follow a path beyond science, would he reject an inquiry because it is unscientific.

While quantum orthodoxy denies that its mathematical formalisms tell us anything about an actual quantum reality, others have disagreed. In 1932, John von Neumann looked at the problem confronted by quantum mechanics if the Schrödinger equation does realistically describe phenomena before they are measured. Because the measuring apparatus, as a physical system, would be described by quantum mechanics, its interaction with a quantum system would proceed quantum mechanically as a superposition of waves propagating deterministically in hyperspace. At some point, the quantum wave function collapses probabilistically and the measuring apparatus is read classically. Mysteries surrounding this "collapse" constitute the "measurement problem." Recognizing that "experience only makes statements of this type: an observer has made a certain (subjective) observation; and never any like this: a physical quantity has a certain value," von Neumann analyzed the chain of events from the quantum system to the measuring apparatus, to the retina, and into the interior of the brain. Further, it is "a fundamental requirement of the scientific viewpoint—the so called principle of the psycho-physical parallelism—that it must be possible to describe the extra-physical process of the subjective perception as if it were in reality in the physical world—i.e., to assign to its parts equivalent physical processes in the objective environment, in ordinary space." The problem is that no one knows how to describe the extra-physical processes of subjective perception in physical terms along the chain of events from the retina to the interior of the brain and therefore the boundary between the observed and the observer is arbitrary. The danger of this arbitrariness, in von

Neumann's opinion, is that it threatens to violate psychophysical parallelism.

In 1939, giving consciousness the upper hand over psychophysical parallelism, Fritz London and Edmond Bauer explicitly espoused the view that consciousness collapses the wave function without specifying the neural events associated with the collapse. In 1963, Eugene Wigner expressed his support for this solution to the measurement problem of quantum mechanics, but later retracted it as it seems to imply solipsism.

An even more radical approach toward solving the philosophical conundrums posed by quantum mechanics was proposed, separately, by Wolfgang Pauli and Erwin Schrödinger. They proposed a synthesis between ancient mystical traditions and modern science.

Pauli called for "a synthesis embracing both rational understanding and the mystical experience of unity," that would be achieved when "natural sciences will out of themselves bring forth a counter pole in their adherents, which connects to the old mystic elements."

Schrödinger warned, "The scientist subconsciously, almost inadvertently, simplifies his problem of understanding Nature by disregarding, or cutting out of the picture to be constructed, himself, his own personality, the subject of cognizance." This objectification is basis of natural science. "But it leaves gaps, enormous lacunae, leads to paradoxes and antinomies, whenever, unaware of the initial renunciation, one tries to find oneself in the picture or to put oneself, one's own thinking and sensing mind, back into the picture." Schrödinger recommended "a bit of a blood-transfusion from Eastern thought," but warned, "we must beware of blunders—blood transfusion always needs great precaution to prevent clotting. We do not wish to lose the logical precision that our scientific thought has reached…"

Max Planck, who, in a self-described "act of desperation" to explain blackbody radiation, introduced the eponymous constant and thereby reluctantly overturned classical physics, wrote, "I regard consciousness as fundamental. I regard matter as derivative from consciousness."

Juan Miguel Marin's 2009 paper, "'Mysticism in Quantum Mechanics: The Forgotten Controversy" contends that Schrödinger's 1950s papers marked the end of quantum mechanics' mysticism controversy, which he interprets largely as the assigning of a role for consciousness in material reality. However, the relationship between mysticism and quantum mechanics—with "mysticism" understood either as consciousness or as the apprehension of the Absolute beyond the limits of the intellect or sensory perception—has not been forgotten.

It has been suppressed in academia, popularized and distorted by the media, and revisited by a few maverick scientists.

The Copenhagen Interpretation, which set aside ontological investigations of quantum reality as empty metaphysics, became the textbook standard: "If I were forced to sum up in one sentence what the Copenhagen Interpretation says to me," said David Mermin (although often attributed to Richard Feynman), "it would be 'Shut up and calculate!'" What Feynman actually told his students at Caltech, using a mixed metaphor, was "Don't ask how it can be like that. You'll fall down the rabbit hole into a blind alley."

Given the remarkable success of quantum mechanics and the rigid and rigorous preparation that prepares and certifies the student to practice his profession, it is not surprising that few have been motivated to explore for cracks in the theory's foundation. Synthesizing quantum mechanics with special relativity physicists predicted the shift of the spectrum of the hydrogen atom caused by virtual particles created and annihilated in the physical vacuum, the Lamb shift, with an accuracy that Richard Feynman once compared to measuring the distance between New York and Los Angeles to within the width of a hair. The paranormal properties of quantum effects have been harnessed to create quantum technologies such as computers that replace binary bits with qubits consisting of superpositions of "0" and "1," quantum cryptography that can transmit "unhackable" codes, and quantum imaging that can take pictures of objects with which it did not interact.

Nevertheless, some physicists have looked outside the confines of quantum orthodoxy for answers. Sir Anthony Leggett, the 2003 Nobel Prize winner for his work on macroscopic quantum coherences, once confessed:

> Occasionally at night, when the full moon is bright, I do what in the physics community is the intellectual equivalent of turning into a werewolf: I question the Universe ... I am inclined to believe that at *some* point between the atom and the brain, it not only may but *must* break down ... I would certainly bet myself that the solution will not be at the level of "inert" physical devices, but would more likely be found at the level of complexity and organization which must be necessary for biology, let alone psychology.

J.S. Bell wrote:

> ORDINARY QUANTUM MECHANICS (as far as I know) IS JUST FINE FOR ALL PRACTICAL PURPOSES ... So it is convenient to have an abbreviation for the last phrase: FOR ALL PRACTICAL PURPOSES = FAPP ... Is it not good to know what follows from what, even if it is not

really necessary FAPP? Suppose for example that quantum mechanics were found to resist precise formulation. Suppose, that when formulation beyond all practical purposes (FAPP) is attempted, we find an unmovable finger obstinately pointing outside the subject, to the mind of the observer, to the Hindu scriptures, to God, or even only to gravitation ... The new way of seeing things will involve an imaginative leap that'll astonish us.

Let us follow that "unmovable finger" and take astonishing imaginative leaps.

Gravity

The path beyond the formulation of quantum mechanics FAPP to gravity has led to the development of new conceptual tools to explore the physical basis of consciousness. Roger Penrose has proposed a solution to the measurement problem according to which gravity collapses the quantum wave function, a process he refers to as objective reduction. He then speculates that the non-algorithmic objective reductions of quantum wave functions in the brain correspond to the non-algorithmic mathematical intuitions that he believes allows mathematicians to transcend the limits imposed by Gödel's theorems by attuning consciousness to the Platonic Realm. Stuart Hameroff then proposed that that "orchestrated objective reductions" of quantum coherent systems of neural microtubules are the physical substrate of Penrose's theory of mathematical intuition.

These speculations are problematic not only because of their reliance on Platonism and the connection between quantum mechanical events in the brain and independently existing mathematical abstractions, but also because quantum effects in the brain are thought to rapidly decohere in warm noisy environments such as the brain. Therefore, they would not influence classical neural events. Nevertheless, there is theoretical and empirical support for the possibility of nontrivial quantum effects in the brain.

Herbert Fröhlich hypothesized that metabolic energy can excite dipoles in neural membranes to coalesce into macroscopic quantum condensates. Hiroomi Umezawa hypothesized that spontaneous symmetry-breaking of quantum fields creates macroscopic quantum effects in the brain. Henry Stapp, a former collaborator with Pauli and Heisenberg, has proposed that the Zeno effect, the continuous observation of a quantum system that prevents its collapse, can prevent decoherence. Recent developments in quantum information, and quantum feedback and control in open systems, have led to new understandings of how quantum coherence can be created and maintained in biological systems. The discovery of quantum coherences in photosynthetic systems and experimental support for quantum coherence in ion channels, the olfactory system, the avian compass, and the retina has lowered the barriers of skepticism.

In 2015, Henry Fisher proposed that nuclear spins of phosphorus atoms could maintain robust quantum coherence in the brain. Fisher first became interested in possible quantum effects in the brain after the symptoms of his intractable depression were relieved by medication. After learning that different isotopes of lithium have different psychotropic effects, he concluded that the difference in quantum spins between the two isotopes was the determining factor. Conventionally, chemical effects at the neural synapse are thought to be the mechanism of action of psychotropic drugs. But lithium isotopes have the same chemical properties. They differ in their nuclear spin, a quantum mechanical property. Further evidence that quantum effects are responsible for the psychotropic effects of drugs is that psychedelic activity is related to the energy of the molecule's highest electron orbitals rather than its binding affinity to serotonergic receptors.

Fisher proposes that phosphorus atoms can maintain robust coherence and entanglement by forming clusters of nine calcium ions and six phosphorus ions, known as "Posner molecules." He speculates that these clusters can be protected from decoherence for days.

Another conceptual tool that has been developed along the path beyond quantum mechanics FAPP to gravity is the Holographic Principle, according to which the universe can be encoded in lower dimensions. A thought experiment performed by Jacob Beckenstein inspired it. Imagining the release of a photon into a black hole, he showed that the entropy of the hole is proportional to its surface area of the hole and therefore units of information are equivalent to Planck areas, $(10^{-35})^2$ meters. This idea led to a holographic model of the universe according to which the three-dimensional observable universe is encoded by Planck area pixels on its two-dimensional surface. These ideas were incorporated into string theories that open the door to the possibility of encoding the universe in one dimension. Beckenstein, pondering the implications of the Holographic Principle asked, "Could we, as William Blake memorably penned, 'see a world in a grain of sand,' or is that idea no more than 'poetic license.'"

Taking these speculations to their ultimate limit, David Bohm posited an implicate order that holographically encodes consciousness and transcendent realities beyond space and time. Karl Pribram developed a holographic model of brain. Likening the resonances of dendritic fields in the sensory cortex to the strings of a piano, he proposes that they are mathematically equivalent to what Dennis

Gabor, the inventor of holography, called a "quantum of information." Operating within a spectral domain, dendritic fields encode images holographically. Frontolimbic excitation shifts consciousness toward a more timeless, holistic, spiritual perspective that characterizes esoteric traditions.

If we examine the Planck level of reality under an even higher magnification, we find spacetime itself flickering in and out of existence during the 10^{-44}-second intervals defined by Planck units of time, giving us fleeting glimpses of eternity. The spacetime continuum is not continuous. Transtemporal threads weave themselves through the gaps in the fabric of spacetime.

Quanta as mathematical abstractions, ghost waves, superpositions of possibilities, clouds of probability engaged in spooky entanglements in hyperspace, Planck area pixels of information, and transtemporal realities feel more like consciousness than ion flows through neural membranes or neurotransmitters crossing synapses. However, the connection between quanta and consciousness is tenuous. Nevertheless, while physicists have justifiably been skeptical of purveyors of New Age "quantum woo" and "quantum flapdoodle," they often throw out the baby with the bath water. The possibility of amplifying quantum effects by creating macroscopic quantum systems could lead to new physical models of consciousness that integrate classical neural effects with quantum effects.

Mind of the Observer

Consciousness has speculatively touched upon quantum mechanics not only as the source of the random collapse of the wave function and as the product of gravitationally induced orchestrated collapses of quantum coherences in neural microtubules but also as an explanation of free will. Taking the idea that consciousness collapses the wave function a step further than von Neumann, or London and Bauer, some scientists have proposed that consciousness can make a choice among quantum probabilities in the brain and thereby explain free will without violating conservation laws. During the 1980s, Sir John Eccles and Friedrich Beck showed how the exocytosis of neurotransmitters from synaptic vesicles could be triggered by quantum events operating within the 5-nanometer vesicular membrane during the one millisecond of delay of synaptic transmission. They proposed that volitional actions can be initiated by choosing which quantum mechanical triggers are pulled. For example, by selectively releasing neurotransmitters in the premotor cortex we can freely choose our actions. Others, such as Robert Jahn and Dean Radin, have proposed that consciousness can telekinetically influence external quantum events.

Alternatively, it is possible that consciousness does not collapse the wave function. Instead, it might preserve and promote quantumness. Stuart Kaufmann has proposed that there is a "poised realm" between the quantum and classical worlds wherein consciousness could preserve and promote quantumness.

While most physicists believe that the probabilities predicted by the equations of quantum mechanics represent the final limit of objective knowledge, in 2016 Adrian Kent, a professor of quantum physics at the University of Cambridge, opined, "I would give credence of perhaps 15% that something specifically to do with consciousness causes deviations from quantum theory, with perhaps 3% credence that this will be experimentally detectable within the next 50 years."

The possibility that consciousness can affect quantum biophysical events in the brain confronts us with a question about the nature of the agent of such causation. Roger Sperry endorsed a theory of emergent interactionism according to which a casual agent emerges from material processes in the brain. Rejecting the undelivered promises of "promissory materialism," Eccles concluded that humans are endowed with divinely created souls.

Wilder Penfield's experiments on awake neurosurgical patients dissuaded him from his earlier materialism and convinced him that "something else finds its dwelling place between the sensory complex and the motor mechanism, that there is a switchboard operator as well as a switchboard." But whether it is a divinely created soul or an emergent causal agent, he could not say.

As a young man, he artistically represented his belief in materialism by painting, on a boulder in his garden, a picture of the brain followed by an equal sign and the word *nous* (mind). However, two critical experiments led Penfield to question his materialist beliefs. One, as mentioned above, involved stimulating the motor cortexes of awake neurosurgical patients. These patients never had any doubt that Penfield's electrodes produced their movements. Another experiment involved electrical stimulation of the temporal lobe. One astonished patient exclaimed that he was aware simultaneously of lying on the surgical table while at the same time he vividly recalled laughing with his cousin in South Africa.

Penfield wondered about the "Self," the "I" who observed these two streams of consciousness. Why was it unaffected by his electrodes? "Where," he wondered, "is the subject, and where is the object if you are operating on your own brain."

After a lifetime of operating on brains and thinking hard about the mysteries of consciousness, the elderly, frail neurosurgeon had doubts about his equation. One cold winter day, he trudged through the virgin snow out to the boulder with a can of paint. When he'd finished what he'd come out to do, a large, freshly-painted question mark had been added to the rock above the equation.

Hindu Scriptures

The path beyond quantum mechanics FAPP to Hindu scriptures and God, adumbrated by Schrödinger and Pauli, is almost universally disparaged by scientists as pseudoscientific nonsense. However, a small number of physicists, such as the Fundamental Fysiks Group out of Berkeley, California, did follow that path. In 1974, a member of the Group, Fritjof Capra, while sitting on the beach under the influence of what Carlos Casteneda had referred to as "power plants," "suddenly became aware of [his] whole environment as being engaged in a gigantic cosmic dance." Previously Capra had experienced this reality as "graphs, diagrams and mathematical theories." Then, as he recalls, "As I sat on that beach my former experiences came to life; I 'saw' cascades of energy coming down from outer space, in which particles were created and destroyed in rhythmic pulses; I 'saw' the atoms of the elements and those of my body participating in this cosmic dance of energy; I felt its rhythm and I 'heard' its sound, and at that moment I knew that this was the Dance of Shiva, the Lord of Dancers worshipped by the Hindus." Capra went on to write *The Tao of Physics*, which started a wave of quantum mysticism.

However, the parallels between Hindu scriptures and modern physics proposed by Capra and others have consisted of affinities between the attempts to express ineffable mystical experiences in ordinary language and the attempts to express the unvisualizable mathematical abstractions of modern physics in ordinary language. Also, unlike Schrödinger and Pauli, who envisioned a synthesis of ancient mysticism and modern science, Capra placed them in a complementary relationship.

However, while the parallels between Eastern mysticism and modern physics has thus far been based on a vague affinity between the language of Hindu scriptures and the language of physics used to describe the realities represented by their equations, Capra and others point out that the language used in Hindu scriptures was not a only an attempt to communicate lofty philosophical reflections but an attempt to describe supersensory perceptions as well. What has thus been overlooked by physicists who have pondered the parallels between

Hindu and other Eastern mystical scriptures are the descriptions of the neuroanatomical basis of the supersensory perceptions upon which those parallels are based.

Hindu scriptures describe a "subtle anatomy" whose central feature is a spiritual, sexual, cosmic energy (*kundalini*) that lies dormant at the base of the spine. When activated, via a variety of methods described by yoga, this energy ascends through concentric passageways in the center of the spine which, proceeding from the outermost to the innermost, are the *sushumna*, *Vajra*, and *chittra nadis*. When the *kundalini* ascends to the brain it activates a center known as the *ajna chakra*, often associated with the pineal gland. This activation leads to paranormal powers or *siddhis*. Ultimately, the *kundalini* reaches the *sahasrara chakra* thereby achieving *nirvana*.

Ancient Taoist scriptures describing acupuncture as applied Taoism describe a similar "subtle anatomy," a system of vessels and meridians through which a cosmic energy, *Qi*, flows. Corresponding to the central *nadis* is the governing vessel. Balancing the *Qi* through various disciplines such as *Tai Chi*, *Qigong*, and acupuncture allows one to live in harmony with the *Tao*, the ineffable Absolute.

God

The path beyond quantum mechanics FAPP to God differs from the one taken to Hindu scriptures. The goal of Hinduism is the union of the soul (*atman*) with the eternal, conscious, infinite spiritual core (*Brahman*) of the finite, changing universe and the liberation from the cycles of birth and rebirth (*samsara*). This union, known as *moksah* or *nirvana*, is a state of timeless bliss. *Brahman* is, therefore, also known as *Satchitananda*, the true ground of being, consciousness, and bliss. The goal of the Abrahamic religions is to bring the eternal, infinite, creative, loving presence of God to the finite realm to create a heaven on earth. Contrary to Hinduism's equivalence of personal consciousness, *Atman*, with the eternal, infinite divinity of *Brahman*, which dissolves individuality into the Infinite, Abrahamic religions posit a unity that embraces a multitude of unique infinite souls.

However, while God is not identical with *Brahman* or the *Tao*, *the* central feature of the anatomical basis of knowing Him is. The Kabbalah, an oral tradition said to predate the first Biblical writings, describes it. Corresponding to the *nadis* and *chakras* of yoga, and the vessels and meridians of acupuncture as in applied Taoism, is a dynamic networks of spheres and pathways called the *Sephirot*, the divine image in which man was created. Corresponding to the central *nadis* and the governing vessel is the central pillar of the *Sephirot*.

Corresponding to the *kundalini* and *Qi* is the *Shekinah*, the exiled, inner, female presence of God.

The Kabbalah scholar Charles Ponce, who speculated Kabbalah contains a lost discipline corresponding to *kundalini* yoga, wrote:

> There's an Adam within each of us ... in exile from the Garden. The aim of Kabbalah is the restoration of the divine man in the medium of mortal man ... We are the laboratory ... If one can learn to connect the thread dangling free from the *sephirot* with the thread of one's own being, one may begin the work of restoration.

While descriptions of the *nadis* and *chakras,* the governing vessel, and the *Sephirot* are almost universally dismissed by scientists as fanciful, primitive symbols, it is possible that ancient mystics interocepted neurophysiological processes that are just now becoming accessible to modern technology. *If descriptions of the "subtle anatomy" are based on interoceptions of actual neuropsychological processes, then the kundalini ascending the central nadis, the Shekinah descending the central pillar of the Sephirot, and the Qi circulating through the governing vessel each correspond to a little-known, threadlike structure originating from the center of brain just below the pineal gland and traveling down the central canal of the spinal cord called Reissner's fiber, as perceived by the sensory system lining the fluid filled cavities and passageways of the neurocele that surrounds it.*

The search for the physical basis of consciousness does not follow a delusional line of reasoning. It leads to the quantum biophysics of the brain and the unmovable finger pointing outside quantum mechanics to gravity, consciousness, Hindu scriptures, and God. Reissner's fiber provides a tangible path along which we can explore these realms that are currently known to us only as unvisualizable mathematical abstractions, or, even more remotely, as parallels with symbols and scriptures from a lost age. Unlike quantum biophysical models based on microtubules, synaptic vesicles, or ion channels which would need to operate as an integrated network of trillions of microscopic elements embedded in billions of spiking neurons, a quantum biophysical model based on Reissner's fiber would be based one a single meter-long fiber floating the fluid-filled cavities of the CSF.

Perhaps the final irony will be that the Great Human Irony was not ironic at all. The scientists' search for God leads neither to materialism and atheism, nor quasi-religious scientisms, nor to the hallucinatory voices created by a vestigial remnant of naturally selected random variations of matter, but to God. An unintended legacy of Jaynes's proposal that the earliest references to God were not based on illusions or projection but on description of the contents of consciousness is that it brings attention to the possibility that those contents were not hallucinations but supersensory perceptions of transcendent realities.

Four

Reissner's Fiber

Reissner's Fiber and the Devil

In 2003, reflecting on science's neglect of Reissner's fiber, two historians of neuroscience, Regis Olry and Duane Haines, published an article titled "Reissner's Fibre: The Exception Which Proves the Rule, or the Devil According to Charles Baudelaire." After reviewing the roots and evolution of various terms used by neuroscientists, they concluded that Reissner's fiber is a counterexample to the "never-ending updating of terms that had been coined by various researchers." A line from the nineteenth-century poet's story, "The Generous Gambler," inspired their equating of Reissner's fiber with the Devil: "My dear brethren, do not ever forget, when you hear the progress of lights praised, that *the loveliest trick of the Devil is to persuade you that he doesn't exist.*" These words were spoken by a "preacher more subtle that the rest of the human herd" and the only man ever to frighten the Devil.

In Baudelaire's story, the narrator hypnotically follows a "mysterious Being" to a "subterranean dwelling" among people of "fatal beauty" and magical radiance expressing the "horror of ennui and desire." The Devil regales his guest with stories revealing the secrets of the universe, conversations with God, and the follies of humankind. He confesses that He invisibly attends all scientific meetings to shape the participants' thoughts and opinions while professing that his supreme goal is bring about the "destruction of Superstition."

Olry and Haines's playful metaphor is apt. The continuing neglect of this strategically located structure remains one of the most remarkable stories in the history of neuroscience.

For thousands of years, fishermen had cut off the heads of their catch of the day, but it was not until 1860 that Ernst Reissner observed a translucent thread finer than a human hair in the central canal of a lamprey. In 1863, Karl Kutschin confirmed Reissner's discovery, naming it "Reissner's fiber." Although Reissner had explicitly distinguished the fiber's "constant features" with "the irregular masses which occasionally fill the central canal and have been mentioned by several investigators to occur in the spinal cord in other animals or in man," subsequent investigators, beginning with Stieda in 1868, asserted that the fiber is an artifact. Anatomists at the time—Viault in 1876, Rohon in 1877, Sanders in 1878 and 1894, and Gadow in 1891—were quick to embrace Stieda's skepticism.

Although the first documented observation of Reissner's fiber occurred in 1860, Emanuel Swedenborg, a Swedish mystic and scientist, nearly discovered it one hundred years earlier. In 1730, he had begun a search for the anatomical basis of the soul. Using a combination of intuitions about correspondences between body and soul, geometrical principles, and direct observation, he developed many remarkably prescient ideas about the brain, including the neuron concept, the hierarchical and somatotopic organization of the brain, the localization of higher cognitive functions in the frontal cortex and the functions of the pituitary gland, foramen of Magendie, and the perivascular spaces.

Based on his observation that cerebrospinal fluid pulsations in the fourth ventricle are "contracted into the narrow form of a goose quill" as they approach the uppermost portion of the spinal cord, Swedenborg deduced the existence of the central canal. It was not conclusively observed, however, until a hundred years later.

In 1743, Swedenborg started writing a planned seventeen-volume work, *The Economy of the Animal Kingdom*.

In volume 3, *The Fibre*, he cryptically described a fiber:

> But the nature of the fiber cannot be learned except by the analytic way, that is to say, by the abundant experience from things posterior and phenomena I investigated physically and philosophically all the way to their causes and principles; for it is utterly remote from the perception of the senses, and goes beyond the sphere of anatomy. Here our primary concern is that we may come to the knowledge of the essence and nature of this fibril, for on this knowledge depends the understanding of the phenomena in the whole of this noble kingdom. For even though we know all things, still they are merely effects, for the entire product of the infinite forces flow forth from the potencies and principles of this fibril; and thus we really understand nothing if we are ignorant of this fibril in respect to its quality.

The following year, while on a trip abroad to obtain research material not available in Sweden, Swedenborg had a series of dreams and spiritual visions. He claimed the Lord had opened his spiritual eyes and commanded him to reveal the inner spiritual essence of His Word. Only by awakening our spiritual sense would the divinity of the Bible be known. He concluded that the Bible describes a rebirth or regeneration of humanity from a material to a spiritual being.

Although wary of being seen as "ridiculous" or dishonest, Swedenborg refreshed his knowledge of Hebrew and began writing *Secret of The Heavens*. Swedenborg's foreshadowing of Reissner's fiber remained in the misty borderland between mystical visions, philosophical speculation, and anatomical observation until 1860.

In 1876, a twenty-year-old medical student, Sigmund Freud, stood poised to remove the scales from the eyes of the investigators who denied that the fiber that appeared before them was really there. Under the direction of Ernst Brucke, a stern, uncompromising individual whose Institute of Physiology was an important part of the materialist Helmholtz School of Medicine, Freud began investigating another of Ernst Reissner's discoveries, Reissner's cells.

As science continued its search for answers to age-old questions about the relationship between man and God, Brucke undertook a study regarding whether the human nervous system evolved continuously from primitive mollusks and fish. His goal was to confirm the Darwinian notion that humans differ from fish and mollusks only by the number of cells and the complexity of their connections.

Each morning Freud gathered specimens from an outside shed. Then, after drawing water from a well in the yard, he descended to his basement cubicle and, by the light of a spirit lamp, carefully dissected, prepared, and studied Reissner's cells, a peculiar, large type of nerve cell located in the spinal cord of the same species of lampreys in which Reissner had discovered the eponymous fiber. Gazing through his microscope, he traced the migration of embryonic stem cells along the inner surface of the hollow tube running through the center of the embryo. Less than a millimeter away, sending filaments toward those cells, is Reissner's fiber.

Freud's investigations led to his first scientific paper in which he concluded: "Reissner's cells are nothing else than spinal ganglion cells which, in those low vertebrates where the migration of the embryonic neural tube to the periphery is not yet completed, remain in the spinal cord."

Freud was a keen observer and an accomplished neuroanatomist. According to his biographer, Ernst Jones, Freud "narrowly missed world fame in early life through not daring to pursue his thoughts to their logical—and not far off—conclusion." Having shown the anatomical continuity between the nerve cell body and the axis cylinders, Freud was "trembling on the very brink of the important neuron theory, the basis of modern neurology."

In the summers of 1879 and 1881, Freud continued his research in Brucke's laboratory and made another important contribution to neuroanatomy. Investigating the internal structure of nerve cells and fibers, he observed lacy networks of fibrils and speculated that they might conduct signals. Electron microscopy would later confirm that Freud was looking at microtubules.

Freud almost certainly became aware of Reissner's fiber during his studies of Reissner's cells. Peering into his microscope, he would have seen the glistening thread. Freud had read Ernst Reissner's papers that described the fiber and communicated with Kutschin and Stieda who were sparring over the nature of the fiber. However, the fiber, as Freud presumably concluded, is not a nerve, and therefore became invisible to him. He never mentioned Reissner's fiber in his neuroanatomical articles or his medical school thesis about the spinal cord of fish as the fiber continued to persuade scientists that it didn't exist.

In the spring of 1899, Porter Sargent, a twenty-seven-year-old doctoral candidate at Harvard, sat examining lengthwise sections of the spinal cord of a lamprey. Curious about the thread-like structure he saw within the central canal, he searched the scientific literature and was astounded that "so peculiar and conspicuous a structure as Reissner's fiber, which is of so great importance in the nervous anatomy as to persist throughout the vertebrate series, should've remained so little known for forty years after its discovery." Similarly, he was dismayed that the ventricles, their lining and content, had been almost entirely dismissed. Sargent set out to disprove the consensus that Reissner's fiber was an artifact.

That same year, Studnicka also concluded that Reissner's fiber is a biological structure in the central nervous system. Contrary to Sargent, however, he believed that the fiber is formed by secretions from cells lining the central canal, comparable to the crystalline style, a translucent rod found in the digestive tracts of bivalves and gastropods. In 1900, he made the first detailed anatomical studies of the subcommissural organ, an ependymal structure located below posterior commissure, a bundle of nerve fibers located along the upper dorsal aspect of the cerebral aqueduct connecting the right and left pretectal areas, but failed to correctly identify it as the main source of Reissner's fiber.

For six years, Sargent devoted himself to investigating the fiber in nearly one hundred species of fish, focusing on species in early stages of evolutionary and embryological development. He laid the foundation for the modern anatomical understanding of Reissner's fiber as a biological structure that runs from the subcommissural organ through the third and fourth cerebral ventricles and central canal and terminates in a dilation at the end of the central canal called the terminal ventricle.

Based on his conclusion that Reissner's fiber links the visual and motor pathways, Sargent proposed that it is a "short circuit" for transmitting "optical motor reflexes" which conferred an advantage in the Darwinian struggle for survival. To support his hypothesis he experimented with a species of small shark, *Squalus acanthia*. He severed Reissner's fiber by inserting a needle probe through a small incision in the sandpapery skin, the cartilaginous skull, and the dural membrane covering the fourth ventricle through which the fiber ran. Closing the incision, he placed the sharks in large circular tanks and observed their avoidance of a wooden oar placed in their path. Comparing the behavior of sharks that underwent a sham operation that involved making an identical incision but not severing the fiber, Sargent observed that the sharks whose fibers were severed had slower responses. His observations of poorly developed Reissner's fibers in kittens and mouse pups, who are born blind, also supported his hypothesis.

Curiously, Kalberlah (1900) and Streeter (1903) continued to agree with previous erroneous characterizations of the fiber as cellular debris or coagulated proteins in the cerebrospinal fluid (CSF). In 1905, William Kolmer's studies of *amnocoetes* (the larval stage of lampreys) prompted him to reject Sargent's characterization of the fiber in support of Studnicka's hypothesis that the fiber is formed by ependymal secretions.

Sargent published his last paper dealing with Reissner's fiber in 1905, a 105-age manuscript titled, "The optic reflex apparatus of vertebrates for short-circuit transmission of motor reflexes through Reissner's fiber; Its morphology, ontogeny, phylogeny, and function. Part 1. The fish-like vertebrates" in the *Bulletin of the Museum of Comparative Zoology at Harvard University*. Sargent concluded his 1905 paper by saying, "The conclusions and the discussion of the results and bearings of this research are reserved for the second part of this paper dealing with the higher vertebrates. This is already well advanced, and it is hoped will appear in about a year."

However, Sargent never published the second part of his paper. He abruptly abandoned his academic career and went on to spend the next decade traveling the globe, "re-educating myself and others, studying and interpreting peoples, their arts and religions." He became a well-known iconoclast writing essays about education and politics, and poetry.

Sargent overcame the devil's trick of persuading scientists that Reissner's fiber doesn't exist. He established the modern basis of its anatomy as a neural structure that runs from subcommissural organ, directly below the pineal gland, through the third and fourth ventricles and central canal to the terminal ventricle. However, Sargent paid a price for his victory over the devil.

Sargent reportedly abandoned his research after a contentious defense of his thesis. Rather than defend the still unknown ideas about the fiber that Sargent was about to publish, Sargent chose to leave the battlefield. In his words, he "shook the dust from Cambridge" and left the university that "had nearly ruined [him] for life."

Hints of Sargent's vanquished dreams appear in his later writings. In works such as *Mad or Muddled, New Immoralities,* and *Is Poetry a Secretion?* he wrote:

> Those who don't conform are abnormal. We have various names to apply to them and supposedly appropriate places in which to sequester them. And it's only the occasional insane man we accept as a genius. But to win plaudits, instead of a padded cell, he must have a good publicist. ... Once in a blue moon, some crank member of a tribe points out something right at hand which no one's seen before. He is greeted by ridicule. Sometimes, they kill him. But eventually the whole tribe sees, too, and then they worship him. History repeats itself.

In 1934, inspired by the majestic power of a lightning storm, he wrote:

> Till I can express myself,
> Until I can set the ether vibrating with my thought,—
> And make the kilocycles sing with my emotion,
> Till I am attuned to each and every fellow
> And speak to them in a common language,
> Till I can twang upon the ether waves as harpstrings
> So that every soul responds,
> I am not free.

Porter Sargent's final publication in 1950 was titled *Is Poetry a Secretion?* The title's allusion to brain activity was as near as Sargent would come to divulging his youthful incarnation as a serious scientist.

To see if I could find any traces of Sargent's promised paper dealing with the significance of Reissner's fiber for higher vertebrates, I contacted Porter Sargent Publishers, Inc., a Boston-based firm, founded by Sargent, which published an education-related list, including a directory evaluating private schools. They were continuing Sargent's legacy of "removing the scales from the eyes" of those who are "miseducated, misled, and misinformed."

The company's president, recalling a 1939 article in *Time* magazine that "the attic in his family home was probably filled with ten tons of papers, his garage with twenty," raised my hopes. At the time of my inquiry, Sargent's daughter, a blind law student, was living there. She graciously arranged to have several boxes of her grandfather's scientific papers delivered to the Porter Sargent Publisher's office.

Sifting through Sargent's scraps and doodlings on loose papers, envelopes and hotel receipts, I read hundreds of handwritten notes about Reissner's fiber. There were also astute, prescient speculations about the mechanism of nerve conduction. Notes from as long ago as 1900 percolated with ideas about ions, membranes, and electrical charges.

I found a handwritten draft of Sargent's last scientific paper with its promise of a well-advanced sequel. But there was not a trace of it.

Reissner's Fiber After Porter Sargent

For several years following his hasty, bitter departure from the scientific community, Sargent's hypothesis that Reissner's fiber is a novel pathway for high-speed transmission of nerve signals was generally accepted. In 1908, inspired by Sargent's research and giving "greatest deference" to his opinions regarding the fiber's function, pioneering neurosurgeon Sir Victor Horsley undertook an investigation of Reissner's fiber in apes. Owing to the fragility of the fiber and its elastic recoil, Horsley was able to examine it adequately in sagittal sections of the spinal cord in only one specimen of *Maccacus cynomolgus*. He showed that the fiber lacked the structure of nerves and did not display Wallerian degeneration. He urged reinvestigation of the fiber before dismissing it as vestigial.

Surprisingly divergent interpretations of what was observed within the neurocele persisted after 1905. In 1908, Howard Ayers reported a "fine-meshed network of fibrils which ... in life practically fills the ventricular cavity." He concluded that these fibrils constitute an "organ of relation bringing all parts of the ventricular cavity into intimate connection." Regarding its function, Ayer hypothesized that it is "connected with control of the ventricular lymph supply and vaso-motor control." Apparently unaware of previous work on Reissner's fiber, Ayers did not mention the fiber in his paper. That same year, Ludwig Edinger, one of the founders of modern neuroanatomy, disputed Reissner's fiber's existence as an actual biological structure.

In spite of the confusing disputes regarding the fiber's status as an actual biological structure following Reissner's initial observations, neuroscientists eventually acknowledged its existence. Unable to disguise itself as cellular debris or an artifact of preservation, the fiber played a new trick to hide from the spotlight of science. In 1909, George Nicholls convinced the scientific community that Reissner's fiber is part of the neural basis of consciousness. Based on his investigations, he concluded that the fiber is an elastic cord that acts as a flexure sensor in fish.

Nicholls disputed Sargent's hypothesis that the fiber transmits signals because Sargent had mistakenly referred to the fiber as an axon. However, the terminology used during the time of Sargent's research to describe fibers in the brain was fuzzy. Due in part to technological limitations, the subtle anatomical differences between Reissner's fiber and axons were unclear. Rudolph Albert von Kölliker, who, in 1845, provided the first proof that axons are extensions of neurons, and who, in 1898, coined the term axon, was unable to decide if Reissner's fiber was an axon, an artifact of preservation, or a "crystallization of biological secretions." When the 1906 Nobel Prize in physiology or medicine was awarded to Ramon Y Cajal and Camillo Golgi, the debate about whether the brain was made of discrete cells or of a continuous web of fibers had not yet been completely settled.

While Sargent did characterize Reissner's fiber as a coalescence of axons, he also distinguished the "axons" that formed Reissner's fiber from "ordinary axis cylinders." He described the fiber as a "highly specialized conduction path" and contrasted the "very thin medullary sheath" surrounding the fiber with the sheath surrounding "ordinary nerves." His description of the fiber as being "anchored" to the sub-commissural organ, like "the inlet of telephone wires into a building," further blurred his characterization of Reissner's fiber as an axon. Given the embryonic status of the term "axon," Sargent's use of the term to describe an hypothesized conduction pathway was justified.

Ironically, Nicholls' ostensible refutation of Sargent's hypothesis was based on his own mischaracterization of the fiber as a "coalescence of cilia-like processes springing from cells," mostly from the sub-commissural organ, but from other ependymal cells lining the central canal as well. He went on to describe the fiber as a "thread of protoplasm" whose mode of contraction is "paralleled only in the scarcely modified protoplasm which forms the stalk of certain Protozoa."

The coiling of the end of the fiber, which Studnicka had observed, was explained away by Nicholls as an artifact resulting from accidental severing of the fiber. He claimed that the fiber ends in an amorphous mass and gave it the inglorious name, "terminal plug."

In 1909, Dendy proposed that the fiber is a strand of connective tissue which transmits changes in its tension to sensors in the subcommissural organ to regulate the flexure of fish. He expressed the hope that the apparently insuperable obstacles standing in the way of experimentally confirming his hypothesis could be overcome.

The following year, Nicholls discovered that Reissner's fiber extends through a pore at the end of the terminal ventricle. Here only skin and a thin layer of connective tissue surround the fiber. Based on his discovery, Nicholls developed a surgical procedure for severing the fiber in live fish and tested Dendy's hypothesis. He concluded that Dendy was correct. However, in 1917 Hovey Jordan replicated Nicholls' experiments and concluded his hypothesis was incorrect. Concerned about uncertainties surrounding the future of his studies at the Bermuda Biological Station for Research, Jordan published his preliminary results and wrote about his plans to investigate the function of Reissner's fiber. His subsequent and final paper about the fiber, which identified the fiber in a ray and trout, offered no suggestions about its function. Reissner's fiber drifted to the backwaters of science.

While Nicholls' misinformed characterization of the fiber as an elastic cord that acts as a flexure sensor in fish has become a little known footnote in the history of Reissner's fiber, his distinction between the fiber and axons has allowed the fiber to play its role as the Devil according to Baudelaire. After Luigi Galvani's eighteenth-century postulation of "animal electric fluid" was shown in 1902 by Julius Bernstein to be ionic flows across semipermeable neural membranes, Reissner's fiber was neglected because it lacked such a membrane.

In 1954, Masashi Enami published his discovery, documented with microphotographs, of a branch of Reissner's fiber across the third ventricle from the hypothalamus to the subcommissural organ in an eel. Puzzlingly, Enami characterized this branch of the fiber as a "coalescence of axons." However, while this branch of the fiber is clearly not axonal, Leatherland and Dodd have shown a connection between the secretory activity of the hypothalamus and the subcommissural organ. Immunoreactions against proteins in found in the fetal human subcommissural organ have been demonstrated in the hypothalamus.

In 1954, Enami also discovered a caudal neurosecretory system located in the piscine equivalent of the terminal ventricle, the urophysis. Injecting extracts from the urophysis into fish and observing their behavior, he concluded that the active component influences sexual behavior and buoyancy. Enami was poised to identify Reissner's fiber as a novel pathway interconnecting its endpoints; the hypothalamus, the subcommissural organ, and the caudal neurosecretory system. However, in 1958, Enami died in a car accident en route to a symposium where he was to have presented a paper. In 1965, Howard Bern isolated the substance Enami had discovered. It was found to be a potent constrictor of blood vessels and named urotensin. While human urotensin has been identified, the terminal ventricle has not been confirmed as a source. Urotensin acts on the habenula which regulates the neural circuits of dreams and those involved in the conditioning of our behaviors by rewards and punishments.

In 1972, Professor Charles Loeser, Department of Anatomy, University of Connecticut Medical School, and I observed previously unreported circular clusters of cells characteristic of secretory systems surrounding the terminal ventricle in a specimen from a human spinal cord. This observation was confirmed and developed during the 1980s by two Russian scientists, A.P. Bakhtinov and P.A. Motavkin, who found that the highest secretory activity coincides with the greatest activity of the human reproductive system. They coined the term intraspinal organ. Their research was abandoned due lack of funding. My team of scientists is currently investigating the terminal ventricle using innovative technologies.

Because Reissner's fiber transports a class of proteins known as spondins that are involved in neurogenesis, and axonal growth and guidance, and because of the fiber's intimate association with the neural stem cells along the ventricular border and with the extracellular matrix, the fiber is thought to play a key role in the embryological development of the brain. Pasko Rakic injected radioactive thymidine into pregnant monkeys and mice and examined the embryonic brains of the offspring. Because thymidine is incorporated only in dividing cells, Rakic was able to trace their development. He discovered and named the "subventricular zone" lining the walls of the cerebral ventricles as the site of origin of all neurons of brain and showed that the subcommissural organ marks the embryological boundary between the motor-sensory area (chordencephalon), and analyzer-correlator areas of the brain (acrencephalon). Reissner's fiber is strategically located because it originates from the subcommissural organ, which marks the embryological boundary between the motor-sensory area (chordencephalon), and analyzer-correlator areas of the brain (acrencephalon).

Under an electron microscope, the 2-micron diameter fiber appears as parallel 5–10 nanometer filaments embedded in a complex matrix. Spaces within this matrix material contain tiny spheres surrounded by a tri-layered membrane filled with an homogenous, granular substance. Extending from Reissner's fiber to the surface of the neurocele are numerous filaments. The fiber's rate of growth correlates with photoperiods and the activity of the pineal gland as measured autoradiographically following the injection of the radioactive isotope S^{35}, which were incorporated into the cysteine-rich fiber.

The function of Reissner's fiber is unclear. The subcommissural organ–Reissner's fiber complex regulates fluid and electrolyte balance. It is also involved in neurogenesis and neural development. Lesions of the fiber in developing tadpoles disrupt mitotic rhythms and tail regeneration. Extracellular matrix (ECM) proteins such as SCO-spondin and F-spondin, potent influencers of axonal guidance and neurite outgrowth, help mediate these morphogenetic and neurogenetic functions. Reissner's fiber binds neurotransmitters including adrenaline, noradrenalin, and serotonin. However, without a biophysical model that could integrate this interaction with possible physical correlates of consciousness, researchers have concluded that the fiber is merely a waste disposal system that detoxifies the CSF.

Reissner's fiber's strategic location and relatively simple structure make it an attractive site for empirically exploring several novel neural mechanisms. First, the membrane-bounded spherical bodies within Reissner's fiber that Kohno interpreted as "cell detritus caught among the filaments as they originate from the SCO" might be exosomes. Consistent with this conjecture is the presence of F-spondin within exosomes. During the past 25 years, these endocytic vesicles have been shown to play key roles in epigenetic information transfer, neuronal plasticity, and morphogenesis in the brain. Reissner's fiber, an ever-growing thread traveling through the neurocele, would be a unique delivery system of exosomes. Second, Reissner's fiber's filaments and its extensions to the surface of the neurocele could transmit electrical signals in a manner similar to the way microtubules do via tubulin. Third, the transmission of vibrations by Reissner's fiber might be an instance of the role that such protein vibrations play in neurosignaling elsewhere in the brain.

Reissner's fiber has also been implicated in the pathogenesis of hydrocephalus. In 1982, Dr. D.H.M. Woolam proposed that Reissner's fiber could be a possible site for future neurosurgical treatment of hydrocephalus. Astonished by a case of hydrocephalus in a fifteen-year-old boy, which resulted in his skull becoming as heavy as the rest of his body, Dr. Woollam hypothesized that tension on Reissner's fiber produced by over-production of CSF triggered signals to lower its production. If Reissner's fiber ruptures, then CSF production races out of control. Woollam believed that:

> Studies in years to come will probably show that Reissner's fibre has an important function and that its presence is by no means for purely ornamental purposes ... For years, the CSF has been thought of as occupying space not needed for anything important. It seems extremely likely that it shortly will return to the exalted position it occupied in the 1,700 years of Galenical medicine as something whose constitution and surroundings have great significance in their own right.

While Woolam's expectations regarding Reissner's fiber and the CSF have yet to materialize, subsequent research has confirmed his intuitions about the role of Reissner's fiber in the pathogenesis of hydrocephalus. Animals lacking Reissner's fiber, due to folic acid or B12 deficiency, develop hydrocephalus. Immunological blockade of secretions from the subcommissural organ has been found in infants with congenital hydrocephalus. Resulting CSF turbulence and malformations of the Sylvian aqueduct due to an absence of Reissner's fiber have been proposed as a contributing factor to the disease.

In 1994, in the guest editorial for the *Journal of Near-Death Studies*, drawing on the similarities between the mystical experiences of yogis and kabbalistic mystics and near-death experiencers, I proposed that Reissner's fiber is the neural basis of near-death experiences and that perceptions of the "silver cord" are a variation of perceptions of the "subtle anatomy." Nearing death, as the brain's energy drains centripetally toward its phylogenetically ancient core, the fiber is perceived just as stars appear in a darkening sky. Subsequently, realizing that the incidence of near-death experiences almost certainly exceeds the incidence of Reissner's fiber in near-death experiencers, I have concluded that most near-death experiences are based on perceptions of a virtual fiber.

Reissner's Fiber in Humans

Besides making itself invisible by using the filters of the neuron doctrine, the fiber has exploited its small size, fragility, and concealment beneath layers of skin, muscle, bone, membranes, and brain tissue to evade detection in the human brain. Investigations of human specimens suggest that Reissner's fiber's activity peaks during the fifth month of human fetal development and completely degenerates by birth. Similarly, investigation of the subcommissural organ suggested that it regresses during late fetal development and becomes a vestigial islet by late infancy. Nevertheless, a few "black swans" have been observed. In 1922 Eric Agduhr observed the fiber in a 14-year-old teenager. In 1935 Lucas Keene found evidence of the fiber in an infant.

In 1961 Bosque Gomez observed a fully developed subcommissural organ in a 60-year-old man.

Reissner's fiber could have thus far evaded observation in human adults because of its rapid post-mortem degeneration and inaccessibility. During life, CSF flow produced by cardiac and respiratory rhythms ceases. The rhythmic beating of cilia along the ventricular surface, which keeps the fiber afloat, also stops. Shortly after death, the fiber sinks to the surface of the neurocele where enzymes released by dying cells break it down. Unless the deceased's head were ghoulishly frozen at the moment of death, the fiber could play its devilish trick.

Observation of the fiber in living subjects is also problematic. The third and fourth ventricles are generally accessible to neurosurgeons only via relatively low-resolution fiber optic devices. Current neuroimaging devices such MRI and PET similarly lack sufficient resolution to detect the fiber. The words of the French investigator of Reissner's fiber, Etienne-Jules Legait, from 1942, remain true today: "when its existence is denied, this fact should be carefully analyzed and discussed: one could not take it into account if fixation is uncertain."

What is certain is that the genetic code for Reissner's fiber has been preserved for more than 500 million years. The machinery for producing the fiber is encoded in the human genome. The epigenetic factors that typically switch off the Reissner's fiber genes during fetal development are unclear but the means of controlling those factors are within our grasp.

Circumneurocelic Sensory System

While it is generally assumed that our external sense organs are the only source of percepts, it is possible that Reissner's fiber and the circumneurocelic sensory system surrounding it could generate them as well. The central nervous system's projections to the body's external sensory organs share anatomical features with the brain's inner surface, the lining of the cerebral ventricles, and central canal of the spinal cord, collectively known as the neurocele.

Dimitri Tretjakov was the first to propose that the structures surrounding Reissner's fiber serve a sensory function. In 1913, he hypothesized that the cilia and CSF-contacting neurons surrounding the fiber form a "central sense organ." In 1921, William Kolmer elaborated on Tretjakov's proposal, comparing Reissner's fiber to the gel-like tectorial membrane of the inner ear which lies beneath Reissner's membrane. He named this novel sensory system the "sagittal organ."

The following year, Agduhr, who, together with Kolmer, discovered specialized sensory neurons bordering the central canal (Kolmer-

Agduhr cells), proposed a similar "ependymal sensory organ." He published a 137-page manuscript dealing with this "central sensory organ in vertebrates." However, contrary to Kolmer, Agduhr concluded that Reissner's fiber is not part of this system. He therefore refused to accept the term *saggital organ* and suggested that the synonymous term *median organ* be used instead. Nine years after Agduhr's criticisms, Kolmer published the results of his research on the structure he had named the *saggital organ*. Based on his extensive observations of lizards and snakes —as well as a detailed study of rhesus monkeys—Kolmer rejected Agduhr's criticisms.

The idea of a circumneurocelic sensory system faded into obscurity until new anatomical methods revived it. The cilia along the surface of the neurocele contain photoreceptor molecules homologous to pineal and retinal opsins. A thin layer of 5-nanometer, striated filaments, similar to ependymally-derived cells of the retina are located on the apical surface of the central canal. CSF-contacting neurons include those which project from the dorsal raphe nucleus into the third ventricle, a site of action of LSD and the key neural input to the subcommissural organ, and opiate receptors surrounding the periaqueductal gray area. In addition to cilia and CSF-contacting neurons are various circumventricular organs. These structures, including the subcommissural organ, organum vasculosum of the lamina terminalis, and the pineal gland, lack the normal blood brain barrier, and have a variety of sensory and secretory functions.

Currently CSF-contacting neurons and the circumventricular organs are thought be involved with physiological functions such as osmoregulation, cardiac regulation, hormone regulation, and circadian rhythms. However, the generation of percepts by the circumneurocelic sensory system is consistent with the features it shares with the external sense organs.

Speculations about the nature of the percepts that might be generated by a circumneurocelic sensory system encounter an impasse elucidated by formidable philosophical arguments against physicalism. As Thomas Nagel famously argued, physical knowledge of a bat's sonar system would not give someone knowledge of "what it is like to be a bat." Similarly, Frank Jackson illustrated the limits of physicalism with the example of a neuroscientist, "Mary," whose knowledge of the world comes exclusively from a back and white television monitor. No amount of neurophysiological knowledge would provide Mary with the subjective experience of knowing the world using a color television monitor.

Although we cannot know what is like to have our circumneurocelic sensory system activated by Reissner's fiber, if the correspondences between the "subtle anatomy" and the Reissner's fiber apparatus are based on interoceptions, then some percepts share visual and proprioceptive pathways with the external sensory system. This would explain how ancient mystics "discovered" Reissner's fiber thousands of years before it was "discovered."

Reissner's fiber's stimulations of the circumneurocelic sensory system could also open new doors of perception. The triggering of our external sensory neurons generates our immediate phenomenal awareness. Triggerings of the circumneurocelic sensory system could generate neural activity commensurate with the neural activity correlated with our ordinary phenomenal awareness. While experiences correlated with the neural activity generated by the fiber's stimulation of the circumneurocelic sensory system would likely be radically different from ordinary phenomenal experience, because they would involve the circuits that underlie our familiar emotional, cognitive, and sensory experience, they would not exceed the limits of our imagination.

But the identification of Reissner's fiber with the "subtle anatomy" implies an even more remarkable claim. Mystics claim that they can open the doors of perception to supersensory realms beyond logic and empirical evidence, beyond the imagination. We are currently denied access to the quantum world because observation, either by an interaction with consciousnesses or by a purely physical interaction, collapses, decoheres, or splits quantum superpositions into classical realities. Physicists grasp the suprasensory quantum world with mathematics because empirical reality is given to us indirectly via measuring devices and a complex chain of neural events. However immediate, direct consciousness of Reissner's fiber as a macroscopic quantum system realities could produce an "immaculate perception" of the suprasensory quantum world. Contrary to Heisenberg's assertion, we *can* become beings other than we are.

The essential problem for musings about "immaculate perceptions" of the suprasensory quantum world is that such perceptions lie beyond the furthest reaches of our imagination. The Schrödinger wave equation, the ψ-function, represents a superposition of all possible outcomes of measurement of a particular quantum system. The impossibility of imagining an unmeasured quantum system was first pointed out by Einstein in a 1935 letter to Schrödinger attempting to clarify his opinion that quantum theory is incomplete:

> A substance in chemically unstable equilibrium, perhaps a pile of gunpowder that, by means of intrinsic forces, can spontaneously combust, and where the average life span of the whole setup is a year. In principle this can quite easily be represented quantum-mechanically. In the beginning the ψ-function characterizes a reasonably well-defined macroscopic state. But, according to your equation, after the course of a year this is no longer the case at all. Rather, the ψ-function then describes a sort of blend of not-yet and of already-exploded systems. Through no art of interpretation can this ψ-function be turned into an adequate description of a real state of affairs; [for] in reality there is just no intermediary between exploded and non-exploded.

Shortly thereafter, Schrödinger published his famous Schrödinger's cat paper, which, in a letter to Einstein of August 19, 1935, he characterized as "very similar to your exploding powder keg." He called his thought experiment a "burlesque," meant to dramatize the absurdity of quantum theory:

> One can even make quite ludicrous examples. A cat is enclosed in a steel chamber, together with the following infernal machine (which one must secure against the cat's direct reach): in the tube of a Geiger counter there is a tiny amount of a radioactive material, *so* small that although one of its atoms *might* decay in the course of an hour, it is just a probable that that none will. If the decay occurs, the counter tube fires and, by means of a relay, sets a little hammer into motion that shatters a small bottle of prussic acid. When the entire system has been left alone for an hour, one would say that the cat is still alive *provided* no atom has decayed in the meantime. The first atomic decay would have poisoned it. The ψ-function of the total system would yield an expression for all this in which, in equal measure, the living and the dead cat (*sit venia verbo* ["pardon the expression"]) blended or smeared out.

The absurdities illustrated by Einstein's example of exploded and non-exploded gunpowder, or of Schrödinger's dead and alive cat, result from imagining the unobserved quantum object as all the observed possibilities existing at once. However, our imagination is limited because it consists of reproductions and combinations of sensory images. Einstein's 1911 acknowledgment to Besso that his brain was incapable of constructing quanta was literally correct. Non-commuting variables operating in an infinite dimension Hilbert space push the imagination beyond itself. If direct consciousness of Reissner's fiber bypasses the transforming chain of events along the visual pathways of the brain, it could transcend the limits of our imagination.

Speculations about the direct consciousness of "uncollapsed" quanta, like all quantum theories of consciousness, face the problem of decoherence. While the suggestion that quantum coherences could be maintained in the meter long fiber for durations sufficient to generate mystical experiences strains our credulity, recent experiments have shown that the creation of such macroscopic systems is possible.

Quantum cavity electrodynamical systems of feedback and control are currently being used to amplify quantum effects. In these experiments the results of quantum non-demolition measurements that allow successive measurements of a quantum without destroying its quantumness are fed to a computer that signals the injection of electromagnetic pulses into a cavity containing the measured quanta. The resulting control of individual quanta, long thought to be unattainable, is now possible. The barriers to the creation of macroscopic quantum systems, "Schrödinger cats," are technical not conceptual.

Reissner's fiber and the circumneurocelic system surrounding it, operating as an analog of a quantum cavity, is uniquely suited to overcome the technical obstacles in the way of creating sustaining extensive quantum coherence. Photosensors with afferent pathways connected to the most complex information processing system in the known universe, the human brain, could perform non-demolition measurements of biophotons emitted from the fiber. Conservative estimates suggest that the brain operates at 1 exaflop, or a quintillion floating point operations per second, compared to 10 petraflops for the fastest supercomputers. If speculations about quantum computations by microtubules or other neural structures are correct, then current estimates of brain computational power based on action potentials would represent an infinitesimal fraction of its true powers.

Efferent pathways from CSF-contacting neurons could inject electromagnetic signals into the neurocelic cavity and thereby control the quanta comprising the fiber. Such a quantum feedback and control system could operate nonconsciously as a self-organizing quantum-dissipative system or consciously as biofeedback system using information about the fiber provided by neuroimaging devices. Conscious control of the fiber's quantumness could tune the clarity and expansiveness of perceptions generated by the fiber. Not only could the fiber generate percepts, but efferent manifestations of the fiber's quantum coherence could influence quantum fields and thereby produce paranormal effects.

Another expansion of consciousness might be achieved by relativistic conduction through the fiber or through its hollow core. The maximum speed of action potential conduction along myelinated axons is 150 m/sec. Researchers have recently developed hollow optic fibers that operated at 99.7% speed of light, nearly 300 million m/sec. If one's stream of consciousness could be directed through Reissner's fiber's hollow core by the circumneurocelic sensory system, then temporal perception might undergo relativistic effects.

When Einstein's dear friend Michael Besso died in 1955, he wrote the following in a condolence letter to his family: "Now he has departed from this strange world a little ahead of me. That signifies nothing. For those of us who believe in physics, the distinction between past, present and future is only a stubbornly persistent illusion." The present moment leaving behind a vanished past and moving toward a not yet existing future is indeed a "stubbornly persistent illusion." The four-dimensional "block universe" toward which the equations of relativity point, like uncollapsed quantum, lies beyond the imagination. Relativistic conduction through Reissner's fiber could open the doors of perception beyond the imagination.

Mathematical models of time travel might also be realized by Reissner's fiber. Wormholes through the fabric of spacetime, first mathematically conceived as Einstein-Rosen bridges, were thought to be physically impossible. During the 1980s, however, Kip Thorn at Caltech proposed that negative energy produced by the Casmir effect, whereby two mirrors separated by a hairsbreadth cancel out certain wavelengths, could sustain traversable wormholes. The hollow tube running through the center of Reissner's fiber, surrounded by 5-nanometer filament, is well suited to function as a laboratory to explore Casmir effects. Consciousness holographically encoded by a one-dimensional thread ensheathed by Reissner's fiber could time travel through a wormhole sustained by negative energy generated by Casmir effects within the inner walls of the fiber.

Mathematical models of reality reflect a world beyond our sensory experience and even beyond our imagination. Whether macroscopic relativistic quantum systems in Reissner's fiber can expand our consciousness to a direct experience of those realities currently known only as mathematical abstractions is a testable hypothesis. The direct consciousness of the fiber itself would constitute a direct consciousness of the noumenon, known phenomenally as a threadlike strand of glycoprotein.

Five

Is Science a Vestige of the Search for Lost Hallucinatory Gods?

The search for scientific truth, according to Jaynes, is, like religion, actually part of a pervasive nostalgia for the certainty of lost hallucinatory gods. For two millennia, like Arthurian knights searching for the Holy Grail, our ancestors looked to oracles and prophets to recover messages from the lost gods to direct our actions. Now we turn to scientists to recover an "innocence of certainty among the mythology of facts." Truth is a culturally given direction determined by the legacy of vanished gods whose voices were generated by neural machinery created by naturally selected random variations of matter.

The "Great Human Irony," according to Jaynes, is that science's quest for God in Nature led to materialism and atheism. Scientisms such as psychoanalysis, behaviorism, and Marxism filled the spiritual void. The loss of ecclesiastic authority led to pseudoscientific substitutes such as unidentified flying objects bringing authority from other galaxies or having left messages from the gods.

Scientific understanding, according to Jaynes, is based on concrete metaphors. We seek metaphors that are familiar and easy and substitute them for the things we wish to understand: "And the feeling of familiarity is the feeling of understanding."

To illustrate, Jaynes points toward the ancient Greeks who understood thunderstorms as the roaring and rumbling of battling superhuman gods creating the familiar sounds of human battlefields. According to Jaynes, "today we reduce the storm to various supposed experiences with friction, sparks, vacuums and the imagination of bulgeous banks of burly air smashing together," images that are no closer to actuality than fighting gods. Both provide familiar metaphors that give us the feeling of understanding.

However, while there is a gap between our scientific understanding of thunderstorms and their actuality, it *is* smaller than the gap the between roaring and rumbling gods and actual thunder. The current model of lightning based on the accumulation of electrical charge, the ionization of air, the generation of plasma channels, and the sudden thermal expansion that produces shock waves has been confirmed in the laboratory. Spectral analysis of the temperature rise in lightning channels from 20,000 K to 30,000 K within their 50-microsecond existence also confirms this model.

Jaynes's belief that all scientific concepts are generated by concrete metaphors is carried to an absurd extreme when he adds charm to his list of metaphors used by physicists along with inertia, impedance, and fields. Charm, the name given to a property of a certain class of quarks, the constituents of hadrons such as protons a neutrons, like other playful labels applied to quarks such as strangeness or flavor, has no metaphorical meaning. It is as meaningless as the name quark coined by Murray Gell-Mann who took it from the nonsense phrase, "Three quarks for Muster Mark" in James Joyce's *Finnegan's Wake*. The true meaning of quarks is rooted in mathematical symmetries such as the organizing of subatomic meson and baryons into octets that Gell-Mann playfully referred to as the Eightfold Way, alluding to the Noble Eightfold Path of Buddhism.

Einstein's Epistemology

An alternative to Jaynes's philosophy of science is Einstein's. For Einstein, scientific truth is a reflection of natural law "which reveals an intelligence of such superiority, that compared with it, all the systematic thinking and acting of human beings is an utterly insignificant reflection." True religiousness is the knowledge "that what is impenetrable to us really exists, manifesting itself as the highest wisdom and the most radiant beauty, which our dull faculties can comprehend only in their most primitive forms." Science for Einstein was a search for God's thoughts.

Scientific understanding, for Einstein, was not based on the substitution of familiar concrete metaphors for things we wish to understand. He sought to grasp reality with mathematics. The truths that Einstein discovered are not based on nostalgia for the lost certainty of hallucinatory gods. They point toward a superior cosmic intelligence before which we stand in "rapturous amazement."

The first step in the creation of a scientific theory, for Einstein, is the creation of axioms. Unlike Jaynes's epistemology, which starts with concrete experience, Einstein's starts with "free creations of thought."

From these axioms, one develops the logically simplest system. What separates such a system from an empty metaphysical system is the empirical confirmation of its predictions.

Tellingly, in contrast to Jaynes's assertion that the conscious search for understanding follows the road of expanding metaphors, Einstein said his conscious search begins at a preverbal level. In a reply to the French mathematician Jacques Hadamard's inquiry about his mental processes, Einstein wrote:

> The words of language, as they are written, do not seem to play any role in my mechanism of thought. The psychical entities which serve as elements of thought are certain signs and more or less clear images which can be "voluntarily" reproduced and combined ... The above-mentioned elements are, in my case, of visual and some of muscular type.

Einstein's first successful application of his epistemology was the theory of special relativity. As a sixteen-year-old, he would imagine himself traveling alongside a beam of light. Common sense told him that he would see a stationary electromagnetic wave, just as a speeding train would appear to be stationary if he were traveling alongside it at the same speed. But Maxwell's equations show that a beam of light couldn't be stationary. It would always be racing away from him at the speed of light, no matter at what speed he was chasing it. The laws of physics must be the same for all observers regardless of their frame of reference.

The laws of physics and common sense battled in his mind. Einstein feared he'd go mad. Something had to give. Ultimately, space and time gave way. The logical forces derived from the axioms that the velocity of light is constant for all observers and the laws of physics are the same in all inertial frames of reference transformed space and time from absolutes to relative variables. The boundary between energy and matter dissolved too, revealing them to be manifestations of the same thing. These revolutions in our understanding were not metaphorical. They are quantitative and empirical.

Ten years after his thought experiment of traveling alongside a beam of light, Einstein had his "happiest thought." While looking out his window, Einstein imagined a painter falling off a roof. The realization that the hapless painter would not feel his own weight became the foundational axiom of general relativity—the principle of equivalence.

Over the next eight years, in an intense effort that threatened his physical health and psychological equilibrium, Einstein created one of the greatest works of genius in the history of humankind—the general theory of relativity. Using non-Euclidean geometries where space curves in higher dimensions and where parallel lines intersect, and tensor calculus, which calculates the paths along a curved four-dimensional spacetime continuum, Einstein redefined gravity as curvatures of a flexible fabric of space and time.

By 1913, Einstein was writing to leading astronomers to persuade them to measure the deflection of starlight by the sun predicted by general relativity. Several expeditions set forth to measure the effect, observable only for several seconds during a solar eclipse, but bad weather and World War I foiled their attempts. On November 18, 1915, when Einstein completed his theory of general relativity, his calculations showed that his theory correctly predicted a tiny variation in the orbit of Mercury. "I was beside myself with joyous excitement," he wrote to his friend. "I felt as if something had snapped inside."

Later, when asked how he'd react if astronomical observations failed to confirm the theory, Einstein quipped, "Then I would have felt sorry for the dear Lord. The theory is correct." Twenty-five years later, he wrote, "the problem of gravitation converted me into a believing rationalist, that is, into someone who searches for the only reliable source of truth in mathematical simplicity."

With an undoubted touch of irony, Einstein said that science begins with the commission of the "metaphysical original sin." First, from the stream of our sensory experience, we "take, arbitrarily, certain recurring sensory experiences" and correlate them with the concept of an independently existing physical object. Second, "we attribute significance to this concept of the bodily object a significance which is to a high degree independent of the sense impressions which originally give rise to it."

The concept of physical reality, Einstein contended, is a free creation of the imagination whose sole utility is that it helps "orient ourselves in the labyrinth of sense impressions." Although Einstein notes that the distinction between "sense impressions" and "mere ideas" is a "necessary prerequisite for scientific and pre-scientific thinking," he asserts, "There is no such thing as a conceptual definition of this distinction (aside from circular definitions, i.e., of such as make a hidden use of the object to be defined). Nor can it be maintained that at the base of this distinction there is a type of evidence, such as underlies, for example, the distinction between red and blue. Yet, one needs this distinction in order to be able to overcome solipsism. Solution: we shall make use of this distinction unconcerned with the reproach that, in doing so, we are guilty of the metaphysical 'original sin.'"

The commission of the metaphysical original sin presupposes the capacity to arbitrarily take certain recurring sense impressions and to correlate them with the concept of an independently existing physical object. It presupposes language that uses nouns. For how else could one grasp concepts from an undifferentiated stream of sensory experience and correlate them with the concept of an independently existing physical object?

Analogous to Einstein's notion of the commission of the metaphysical original sin is Noam Chomsky's theory of the discontinuous evolution from an analog system in which, for example, the continuous varying of the intensity of warning cries could signal whether a tiger was near or far to a digitized system of language. According to Chomsky, this evolutionary discontinuity occurred 100,000 years ago as the result of a chance mutation that produced the neuroanatomical basis of language in "near perfect form." This event was analogous to planting a seed crystal in a supersaturated solution to create a digital infinity.

The nature of that hypothesized mutation and the phenotypical changes in the central nervous that it would have produced remain unknown. The evolutionary transition from the persistence of Reissner's fiber into adulthood to its typical late fetal involution could provide such an explanation. Because Reissner's fiber is active during embryological development, persists into adulthood in rare cases, and is present in our closest ancestors, it is likely that its current typical fetal involution in humans is a recent evolutionary development.

The evolutionary leap from analog language to digitized language not only provided the tools for committing the metaphysical original sin but set humanity on the road of science. Science developed from our dissatisfaction with the lack of logical unity of the primary concepts created by the "metaphysical original sin." To unify the diversity of physical objects such as trees and stones, we create a secondary layer of concepts consisting of imperceptible realities, such as atoms and universal forces that constitute and govern the objects of the primary layer. Einstein believed that this process of unifying our knowledge could proceed until we could "know God's thoughts," and "whether God had any choice in creating the world." He believed in the power of mathematics to grasp reality "as the ancients dreamed."

Impasses on the Road to Truth

While Einstein repeatedly expressed his faith that physics provides a path to know God's thoughts and lift the veil of quantum uncertainty, he pointed to several impasses along the road to Truth. The first impasse occurs when equations explode into infinities. This occurred when physicists followed the equations of general relativity and astronomical observations to their logical conclusion. For two hundred and fifty years, the Newtonian model of an eternal, static universe in which objects follow Euclidean laws of geometry in absolute time and space, a stage that is unaffected by anything external, was the entrenched cosmological paradigm. However, after having followed his "happiest thought" to its logical conclusion, Einstein showed that space and time form a unified continuum that is curved and stretched by matter.

Realizing that his model of the universe is unstable, Einstein introduced a "cosmological constant," a repulsive force to balance gravity. In 1922, the Russian cosmologist Alexander Friedman derived solutions to Einstein's equations that predicted an expanding universe. In 1929, the American astronomer Edwin Hubble observed that starlight is "red-shifted." Like the sound of a train whistle that shifts to a lower pitch as it speeds away from us, light shifts toward the lower, red, end of the spectrum as its source speeds away from us. Therefore, the universe is expanding. In January 1931, after riding up the winding road to Mount Wilson with Hubble in a Pierce Arrow touring car to actually "see" the universe expanding through the telescope, Einstein called the cosmological constant "my greatest blunder." However, it was not until the 1960s, when Penzias and Wilson accidentally discovered the 13 billion year-old echoes of the Big Bang, that the old cosmological paradigm was overturned. Extrapolating backward in time 13.8 billion years, the universe vanishes into an "initial singularity," a fusion of nothingness and infinity devoid of even space and time. The initial singularity is a "place," as Einstein once remarked, that equations describing empirical reality cannot go. We are left to ponder the imponderable question of why there is something instead of nothing.

Infinities also plague quantum field theories. The mathematics used to describe quantum fields, such as the self-interaction of an electron, leads to infinites that can be eliminated only by arbitrarily quantifying one's ignorance in a process called renormalization.

Georg Cantor tried to establish a connection between mathematics and God by developing a hierarchy of infinities. Cantor called the "smallest" infinity, countable numbers, $\aleph_0$, aleph sub-zero. The next level consists of the non-countable numbers, all the points that lie on a line including irrational and transcendental numbers such as the square root of two and pi. He called this rung $\aleph_1$, aleph sub-one. Believing that he was communicating directly with God, Cantor, in a letter written shortly before his death, wrote about "completely individual unity in which everything is included, which is the *Absolute*, incomprehensible to the human understanding. This is the *Actus Purissimus*, which by many is called God." While ridiculed by many of his contemporaries, David Hilbert wrote, "From his paradise that Cantor with us unfolded, we hold our breath in awe; knowing, we shall not be expelled."

The second impasse derives from the uncertainty of mathematics and its relationship to physical reality. Einstein succinctly expressed the problem: "As far as the laws of mathematics refer to reality, they are not certain, and as far as they are certain, they do not refer to reality." The uncertainty of mathematical descriptions of reality arises from the fact that even the most self-evident axioms are free creations and therefore replaceable. Euclid's axiom, for example, that parallel lines never meet or diverge was replaced by the axioms of non-Euclidean Riemann geometry that allows for intersecting and diverging parallel lines. It is the mathematical basis of the curved spacetime continuum. The connection between mathematics and reality is uncertain because the connection between ideas and sensory experience that provides the touchstone for scientific truth, as colorfully expressed by Einstein, is analogous to "check number to overcoat" rather than "soup to beef."

Not only is the axiomatic foundation of mathematical theories subject to change, but there will always be truths that cannot be logically derived from those axioms. Also, the consistency of the system is unprovable. Furthermore, even if the mathematical basis of physics were final and logically certain, the observations that would verify such a system are known to us indirectly along a chain of events from a measuring apparatus, to the eye, to the occipital cortex. As Einstein pointed out to Heisenberg, we cannot claim to have observed anything until that process is understood. However, such an understanding would be based on another observing system whose observations are neural constructions.

Third, there is the paradoxical situation the metaphysical sin has created. In a letter he wrote to Herbert L. Samuel in 1950, Einstein succinctly expressed the paradox:

> In truth, the positing of "Realities" that exist independently of my experience is an aggregate of mental constructions in which, however, we place more intellectual trust than we do in the interpretations that reflect our individual experiences. This explains why our confidence is inspired by such sentences as "There were, trees," even before some living being could perceive them.
> We can thus state a paradox: Reality as we know it exclusively consists of our own fantastical imaginings.

The fourth impasse arises from the stratification of scientific systems toward increasing remoteness from concrete experience. The sole utility of scientific systems of thought, according to Einstein, is that they make our sensory experience intelligible. However, as the scientific image becomes increasingly stratified, the deeper layers become increasingly removed from direct experience. One-dimensional strings and two-dimensional branes vibrating in compacted higher dimensions are unifying concepts reaching out to the primary layer of human thought, familiar, touchable reality. The price paid for logical unity is emptiness of content.

Fifth, Einstein's quest for a universal deterministic theory is paradoxical because the brain, which would create it, would also be bound by deterministic laws. Einstein agreed with Spinoza's identification of the mind and brain. How then could a physicist's brain freely create thoughts?

The final impasse on Einstein's road to know God's thoughts was expressed in a letter to his long-time friend Maurice Solovine:

> You find it remarkable that the comprehensibility of the world seems to me a wonder or an eternal secret. Now a priori, one should, after all, expect a chaotic world that is in no way graspable through thinking. One could (even should) expect that the world turns out to be lawful only insofar as we make an ordering intervention. It would be a kind of ordering like putting into alphabetic order the words of a language. On the other hand, the kind of order which, for example, was created through the discovery of Newton's theory of gravitation is of a quite different character. Even if the axioms of the theory are put forward by human agents, the success of such an enterprise does suppose a high degree of order in the objective world, which one had no justification whatever to expect a priori. Hence lies the sense of "wonder" which increases ever more with the development of our knowledge.

Then, in a revealing passage, he concluded:

> There lies the weakness of positivists and professional atheists who are elated because they feel that they have not only successfully rid the world of gods but "bared the miracles." Oddly enough, we must be satisfied to acknowledge the "miracle" without there being any legitimate way for us to approach it. I am forced to add that just to keep you from thinking that—weakened by age—I have fallen prey to the clergy.

Einstein encountered not only a series of impasses along his road to scientific truth and a final impasse before which he contented himself with feelings of awe and wonder before the miraculous. He also found himself entangled in webs of contradictions within his self-imposed scientific paradise. Einstein believed, "Everything is determined, the beginning as well as the end, by forces over which we have no control. It is determined for the insect, as well as for the star. Human beings, vegetables, or cosmic dust, we all dance to a mysterious tune, intoned in the distance by an invisible piper." However, he also based his cosmic religious feelings on the miraculous power of "free creations" of thought. Similarly, he "consider[ed] ethics to be an exclusively human concern with no superhuman authority behind it." For Einstein, morality belongs to the sphere of religion, invented by moral teachers, and developed along a turbulent road of conquest, oppression, slavery, and genocide. But, unlike scientific truth which reveals a superior mind that represents his conception of God, he replied to a Japanese scholar, "'Religious truth' conveys nothing clear to me at all."

Einstein's Exile from His Religious Paradise

Einstein's characterization of the clergy as victimizers originated from a traumatic episode related in his *Autobiographical Notes*:

> When I was a precocious young man, I became thoroughly impressed with the futility of hopes and strivings that chase most men restlessly through life. Moreover, I soon discovered the cruelty of that chase, which in those years was much more carefully covered up by hypocrisy and glittering words than is the case today ... As the first way out there was religion, which is implanted into every child by way of the traditional education-machine. Thus, I came—though the child of entirely irreligious (Jewish) parents—to a deep religiousness, which, however, reached an abrupt end at the age of twelve. Through the reading of popular scientific books I soon reached the conviction that much in the stories of the Bible could not be true. The consequence was a positively fanatic orgy of free thinking coupled with the impression that youth is intentionally being deceived by the state through lies; it was a crushing impression...

As recalled by his sister Maja, young Albert "heard about divine will and works pleasing to God," and began following a kosher diet and practicing other traditional Jewish observances. Alexander Moszkowski, who, based on personal conversations with Einstein, wrote his first biography in 1920, described how the beauty of nature nourished his religious feelings:

> The pure joy of Nature entered into the heart of the boy ... Nature whispered songs to him, and at the coming of the spring-tide infused his being with joy, to which he resigned himself in happy contemplation. A religious undercurrent of feeling made itself manifest in him, and it was strengthened by the elementary stimulus of the scented air, of buds and bushes, to which was added the educational influence of home and school.

When Einstein began taking violin lessons at the age of six, "He thought out little songs in praise of God, and used to sing them in pious seclusion ... Music, Nature and God became intermingled in a complex of feeling..."

The most influential popular science book that ended young Einstein's religiosity was Ludwig Buchner's *Force and Matter*. Einstein wrote that the core of the conflict between science and religion is the clerical teachings about an anthropomorphic God. The God to whom young Einstein's songs, prayers, good deeds, and observances were directed was surely such a God. Such beliefs, Einstein read in Buchner's book, were an outgrowth of the deification of animals and animal-human hybrids. "If oxen or lions had hands and could paint," said Buchner, quoting from Xenophanes, "they would undoubtedly represent their gods in the form of oxen or lions."

Further distancing young Einstein from his childhood religiosity undoubtedly was the conflict between Buchner's assertion that only eternal matter and force exist and the Biblical account of a beginning. Ironically, Einstein would ultimately, albeit reluctantly, show Buchner's conception of eternally existing force and matter to be false. However, the conflict between a literal interpretation of Genesis and Darwinian evolution was sufficient to crush Einstein's religiosity.

In 1891, at the age of twelve, Einstein abandoned his childhood God and turned to science: "Out yonder, there was this huge world, which exists independently of us human beings and which stands before us like a great, eternal riddle, at least partially accessible to our inspection and thinking ... Similarly motivated men of the present and of the past, as well as the insights they had achieved, were the friends which could not be lost." The road to this new scientific paradise "was not as comfortable and alluring as the road to the religious paradise," but it was trustworthy. Einstein followed that road, in his words, as a "deeply religious unbeliever" inspired by "cosmic religious feelings" as far as he could. While the "clergy" who taught young Einstein childish anthropomorphic conceptions of God might justifiably be perceived as victimizers, there are also "clergy" who form a chain of whisperers transmitting lost secrets from Eden.

Einstein criticized "the fanatical atheists whose intolerance is of the same kind as the intolerance of the religious fanatics ... They are like slaves who are still feeling the weight of their chains which they have thrown off after hard struggle. They are creatures who—in their grudge against the traditional 'opium of the people'—cannot hear the music of the spheres." Nevertheless, Einstein continued to feel the weight of those chains. While he was rapturously attuned to the "music of the spheres," he was deaf to the whispered echoes from Eden.

Spinoza, God, and the Kabbalah

After his faith in the Biblical God of Abraham, Isaac, and Jacob was shattered, Einstein turned to "Spinoza's God, who reveals Himself in the lawful harmony of the world, not in a God who concerns Himself with the fate and the doings of mankind." But Spinoza's relation with his God was different from Einstein's relationship with what he interpreted as Spinoza's God. When questioned by an interviewer whether he believed in Spinoza's philosophy, Einstein replied:

> I can't answer with a simple yes or no. I am not an atheist and I don't think I can call myself a pantheist. We are in the position of a little child entering a huge library filled with books in many languages. The child knows someone must have written those books. It does not know how. It does not understand the languages in which they are written. The child dimly suspects a mysterious order in the arrangement of the books but doesn't know what it is. That, it seems to me, is the attitude of even the most intelligent human being toward God.

Spinoza, in contrast to Einstein, boldly claimed, "The human mind has an adequate knowledge of the eternal and infinite essence of God." Ultimately, we can achieve a "union of the mind with Nature," "the highest good."

Spinoza believed that there is a level of knowledge beyond science called "intuitive knowledge." It "proceeds from an adequate idea of the formal essence of certain attributes of God to an adequate knowledge of the essence of things." The ascent of knowledge, from the fragmentary, confused presentation of reality by our senses, to scientific knowledge, to intuitive knowledge, is a movement towards "knowing the body under a form of eternity." Spinoza asserts that, "Whatever the mind understands under a form of eternity it does not understand from the fact that it conceives the present actual existence of the body, but from the fact that it conceives the essence of the body under a form of eternity … Our mind, in so far as it knows itself and the body under a form of eternity, necessarily has a knowledge of God, and knows it is in God and is conceived through God." The ultimate unity of God and man is expressed in his belief "that God, in so far as he loves himself, loves mankind, and consequently, that the love of God towards men and the mind's intellectual love towards God are one and the same."

Spinoza, like Einstein, harshly criticized the clergy for promoting childish superstitions about an anthropomorphic God and elevating blind faith and obedience above reason. He leveled even harsher criticism at kabbalists:

> Whether they are actuated by folly and infantile devotion, or whether by arrogance and malice so that they alone may be held to possess the

secrets of God, I do not know; this much I do know, that I find in their writings nothing which has an air of Divine secret, but only childish lucubration. I have read and known kabbalistic triflers whose insanity provokes an unceasing astonishment.

The kabbalistic triflings to which Spinoza refers were the attempts find divine secrets from the numerology, typography, and didactical marks in the Hebrew letters of the Torah. One prominent method was gematria, according to which the Torah contains encoded meanings that can be decoded by a variety of methods based on the geometry and mathematical equivalences of Hebrew letters. While Spinoza was contemptuous of gematria and other methods of decoding the Torah, he acknowledged, "Certain Hebrews who seem to have seen, as if through a cloud, that God and God's intellect and the things know by Him are one and the same."

This grudging, vague allusion to kabbalists belies the indisputable fact that Spinoza's philosophy is indistinguishable from kabbalistic philosophy. Abraham Herrera's *Gate of Heaven* first introduced the concepts of the kabbalah to young Spinoza. Herrera tried to distill the obscure, earlier Kabbalah texts so that they would be accessible to philosophers. The similarities between Spinoza's *Ethics* and the Kabbalah, especially Herrera's interpretations, were noted by Jacques Basange and Georg Wachter shortly after its posthumous publication. Indeed, around 1700 when Basange asked a leading rabbi, probably Isaac Aboab de Fonesaca, a student of Herrera, his opinion of Spinoza's works, he replied that Spinoza had plagiarized kabbalistic philosophy.

Scholars, beginning with the late seventeenth century's emphasis on Spinoza's rationalist and anti-religious views, have overlooked the connection between Spinoza's philosophy and the Kabbalah. However, recently they have rediscovered it.

Moshe Idel, the world's foremost Kabbalah scholar, cites two influences from the thirteenth-century ecstatic kabbalist Rabbi Abraham Abulafia. Abulafia used gematria to show equivalence of the Hebrew words for God and Nature: *elohim* = *ha-teba`* = 86. This is the basis of Spinoza's philosophy. He also used the Hebrew expression "*ahabah elohit sikhlit*" ("divine intellectual love"), which foreshadowed Spinoza's expression "*amor Dei intellectualis*," the intellectual love of God. The expression "*ahabah elohit sikhlit*" is repeated by the popular fifteenth-century Maimonidean philosopher, Rabbi Abraham Shalom.

Spinoza was also influenced by the sixteenth-century kabbalist Moses Cordovero, whose words are echoed by Spinoza:

> But the creator is Himself knowledge, the knower and the object known. His knowledge does not arise from His directing His thoughts to things

outside of Him, since in comprehending and knowing Himself, He comprehends and knows everything that exists.

In, *The Influence of Abraham de Hererra's Kabbalah on Spinoza*, Miquel Beltran shows that Spinoza's theory of emanations from the Absolute Infinite, the body under a form of eternity, and God's dependence on humankind's love to love Himself correspond to the Kabbalah's concepts of the *Ein-Sof*, Adam Kadmon, and the role of humankind in repairing the severed connection to God. According to the Kabbalah, the transtemporally eternal absolutely infinite *Ein-Sof* emanated Adam Kadmon, the image in which man, his microcosmic counterpart, was made. His "anatomy" is represented by the *Sephirot*. By following God's commandments and doing good deeds that are pleasing to God we can recreate a new harmony between heaven and earth where God's love for man and man's love for God are one. For Spinoza, the anatomy of Adam Kadmon became the body under a form of eternity that is realized as the body gains activity.

Spinoza says that the prophets were said to "possess the Spirit of God" because the ancient Hebrews were ignorant of the cause their prophetic knowledge. Spinoza also confesses his ignorance as to the "particular law of Nature" which produced prophecy. Regarding the certainty with which prophetic knowledge is proclaimed, Spinoza opines, "ordinary knowledge is no whit inferior to prophetic, unless we believe, or rather dream that the prophets had human bodies but superhuman minds and therefore, that their sensations and consciousness were entirely different from our own." Spinoza mocks this possibility, but if the prophets were extremely rare individuals who possessed fully functional Reissner's fibers, then they may indeed have possessed superhuman minds.

Although Spinoza rejects the idea that prophetic knowledge communicated with words is superior to ordinary knowledge, he contends that "God can communicate directly with man" without "intervention by bodily means." Such knowledge is neither contained nor derivable from natural knowledge and, therefore, necessarily requires a superhuman mind. Such a mind, Spinoza believes, was uniquely possessed by Jesus. According to *Ethics*, Jesus would have known his body "under a form of eternity and therefore have known the eternal infinite essence of God."

Einstein remained deaf to the whispered echoes telling the "secrets of the Old One" that are purported to have originated from the original counterpart to his childhood religious paradise. Although he professed allegiance to Spinoza's God, Einstein stopped short of Spinoza's claim that "Our mind, in so far as it knows itself and the body under a form of eternity, necessarily has a knowledge of God, and knows it is in God and is conceived through God." For Spinoza our mind can unite with Nature. For Einstein we can only dimly perceive an insignificant reflection of Nature. Einstein admired Spinoza's embrace of reason and deterministic natural laws. However, in a response to a request from his friend Siegfried Hessing to write a foreword to his book about Spinoza, Einstein replied, "Unfortunately to like Spinoza is not sufficient to write about him: one must leave to those who have gone further into the historical background." Which, as we have seen, leads to the identification of Spinoza's "body under a form of eternity" with the anatomy of Adam Kadmon.

Ever since his traumatic abandonment of his childhood religious paradise, Einstein's heart and mind battled over his choice to follow the less alluring road of physics. In 1923, when Einstein visited Palestine to support Zionism and to deliver the first lecture at the unfinished Hebrew University in Jerusalem, he met the kabbalist and first chief Rabbi of Jerusalem, Rav Kook. As recounted by the Kook's secretary Rabbi Shmuel Schulman, Einstein and Kook exchanged ideas about the Kabbalah. Schulman recorded that "the Rav related to the comprehensiveness of the professor's method and commented that it is a common sight in ancient Jewish treasures that some wondrous revelation that astounds the whole humanity is found in some hidden corner of our ancient literature." But the concealed connection between Spinoza's God and the Kabbalah remained invisible to Einstein.

When asked to stay in Jerusalem, he responded, "The heart says yes, but the mind says no." When Einstein delivered the inaugural lecture, he was introduced with the words, "Mount the platform which has been waiting for you for 2,000 years." While Einstein rejoiced, "I consider this the greatest day of my life," he later recorded in his diary, after observing Orthodox Jews praying at the Western Wall of the ancient Temple in Jerusalem, "dull-witted kinsmen were praying aloud, their faces turned to the Wall, their bodies rocking to and fro. A pathetic sight—men living in the past, not in the present."

Einstein's ambivalence regarding resonances between his childhood religious paradise and its Biblical roots is also reflected in a curious encounter with Isaac Newton. Upon Newton's death in 1727, a large collection of papers containing over 7,500 handwritten pages with more than eight million words dealing with alchemy, prophecy, and the Kabbalah were, in accord with Newton's wishes, hidden in his niece's home. There, they remained unread for over 200 years until they were auctioned off at Sotheby's in 1936. Newton's annotated, worn, dog-eared copy of Christian Knorr von Ronsenroth's *Kabbalah denudate*, which includes Herrera's distillation of Lurianic Kabbalah, is housed at Cambridge University. His writings refer to the *Sephirot* and Adam Kadmon. Most of Newton's work was devoted to recovering what he called "long lost truths," the *prisca sapientia*, sacred wisdom revealed to Adam and Moses directly by God.

John Maynard Keynes and Abraham Yahuda purchased two of the main collections. After perusing Newton's paper, Keynes remarked, "Newton was not the first of the age of reason, he was the last of the magicians." Explaining this assessment, he said that Newton believed that the universe was a secret riddle that could be read by applying reason to clues that God had left. These clues could be "found partly in the evidence of the heavens and in the constitution of elements (and that is what gives the false suggestion of his being an experimental natural philosopher), but also partly in certain papers and traditions handed down by the brethren in an unbroken chain back to the original cryptic revelation in Babylonia."

Yahuda, the son of a rabbi, searched for Hebrew sources that pre-dated the "cryptic Babylonian revelations." In the late summer of 1940, Yahuda and his wife visited Einstein at his summer retreat at Lake Saranac in the Adirondacks. In letter dated September 1940, Einstein wrote:

> My dear Yahuda,
> Newton's writings on biblical subjects seem to me especially interesting because they provide deep insight into the characteristic intellectual features and working methods of this important man. The divine origin of the Bible is for Newton absolutely certain, a conviction that stands in curious contrast to the critical skepticism that characterizes his attitude toward the churches. From this confidence stems the firm conviction that the seemingly obscure parts of the Bible must contain important revelations, to illuminate which one need only decipher its symbolic language. Newton seeks this decipherment, or interpretation, by means of his sharp systematic thinking grounded on the careful use of all the sources at his disposal.
>
> While the formative development of Newton's lasting physics works must remain shrouded in darkness, because Newton apparently destroyed his preparatory works, we do have in this domain of his works on the Bible drafts and their repeated modification; these mostly unpublished writings therefore allow a highly interesting insight into the mental workshop of this unique thinker.

Newton passionately strived to re-establish the thread from God's revelations to Adam and Moses to the future. He translated the Bible from the original Hebrew. He studied the Biblical descriptions of the floor plan of the Temple in Jerusalem and the blueprint of the

Tabernacle revealed by God to Moses searching for lost secrets. He studied the prophecies of Daniel to calculate the time of the return of the Jews to Israel and the coming of the messianic era. However, because Newton was a mathematician and physicist, his search for "long lost truths" were focused on mathematics rather than the biological basis of those lost truths.

While Einstein had initially encouraged Yehuda to publish Newton's papers, in an interview with the historian of science I.B. Cohen that took place just two weeks before he died, Einstein said that it was significant that Newton had "sealed them all up in a box." Newton had "obviously" not wanted to publish these speculations during his own lifetime. Einstein said, "with some passion," that he hoped they would not now be published.

The consequences of his inability to find an intellectually honest way to stay in his childhood religious paradise continued to follow him. In 1945, Einstein responded to the novel *The Death of Virgil*—started by Hermann Broch in a concentration camp and completed in Einstein's home—by saying, "I am fascinated by your Virgil—and am steadfastly resisting him. The book shows me clearly what I fled from when I sold myself body and soul to science—the flight from the 'I' and the 'We' to the 'It.'"

In any event, Einstein never took the fork in the road of science that would have led back to the kabbalistic roots of Spinoza's philosophy or to the kabbalistic secrets of the *prisca sapientia* that underlie Newton's quest for the secrets of the "Old One." His "grudge against the traditional 'opium of the people'" made him deaf to lost secrets. He feared the "clergy" like the flaming swords guarding the eastern gate of Eden.

About a year before his death, Einstein wrote to Eric B. Gutkind, author of *Choose Life: The Biblical Call To Revolt*, disputing his belief that we can and should assert our free will to align our thoughts and behaviors with God's will as revealed in the Bible.

> The word God for me is nothing more than the product and expression of human weaknesses, the Bible a collection full of honorable but still primitive legends. No interpretation, no matter how subtle, can change it (for me). These subtilised interpretations are naturally highly diverse and have almost nothing to do with the original text. For me, the unadulterated Jewish religion, like every other religion, is an incarnation of primitive superstitions.

However, as Spinoza pointed out, the oldest complete written texts of the Bible are "fragmented" and "mutilated" versions of the original. In *A Theologico-Political Treatise*, he proclaims that he has no wish to deny that the Hebrews who had witnessed the revelations to Moses at Mt. Sinai "witnessed marvels beyond those which happened to any other nation."

Not only is the German translation of the Bible that Einstein refers to as the "original text" a "fragmented" and "mutilated" version of the Bible that was revealed to Moses, or, according to Jaynes, an embellished forgery based on earlier products of the bicameral mind, but the "subtilised interpretations" that Einstein claims have "almost nothing to do with the original text" are, according to Jewish tradition, based on an oral tradition that predates the written Bible. The secrets of this oral tradition were revealed to Moses as the Oral Torah along with the Written Torah. They are the source of the "subtilised interpretations" to which Einstein refers. The "highly diverse" nature of the "subtilised interpretations" with which Einstein was familiar derives from the fact that the oral tradition is even more fragmented and mutilated than the written Bible. It was passed in secret along a chain of elite sages for thirty-four generations. Like the message in a game of Chinese whispers, the first germinal forms of the Oral Torah that were committed to writing by Rabbi Yehuda NaNasi in 189 were distorted, disguised, and embellished.

Not only is the "original text" to which Einstein referred fragmented and mutilated, and the basis of its interpretation distorted, disguised, and embellished, but if Reissner's fiber was the neural basis of the original revelation then we stand before the Bible like aphasics with damaged Wernicke's areas reading Shakespeare. Just as no "art of interpretation" could turn the ψ-function into an adequate description of reality in terms of sensory experience, "no interpretation, no matter how subtle," of the Hebrew letters of the Bible in terms of sensory experience can provide an adequate understanding of realities experienced by the prophets. Rather than having almost nothing to do with the original Bible, the "subtilised interpretations" are its truest, albeit highly distorted, reflection of the original Bible.

The *Zohar*, one of the foundational texts of Kabbalah, warns:

> Woe to the sinners who look upon the Torah as simply tales pertaining to things of the world, seeing only the outer garment ... But the righteous whose gaze penetrates to the very Torah, happy are they. Just as wine must be in a jar to keep, Torah must be contained in an outer garment. That garment is made up of the tales and stories: but we, we are bound to penetrate beyond.

The clergy whom Einstein characterized as victimizers were the "sinners," the literalists who did not penetrate beyond its tales and stories. The identification of the body under a form of eternity and the "subtle anatomy" of Adam Kadmon with Reissner's fiber might provide a tangible path to go beyond the limits of Einstein's epistemology.

1912 Manifesto

In 1912, Einstein and Freud signed a Manifesto that provided a philosophical framework for a possible convergence of physics, neuroscience, psychology, and anthropology upon absolute knowledge:

> The theory of relativity touches upon the most searching questions thus far of epistemology: Is absolute or is only relative knowledge attainable? Indeed, is absolute knowledge conceivable? It comes here directly to the question of man's place in the world, the question of the connection of thought with the brain. What is thought? What are concepts? What are laws? In psychological problems, physics and biology come together. And finally, the anthropological sciences especially history and sociology, find themselves brought into closer and closer connection with biological concepts.

By envisioning the converging paths of the anthropological sciences and biological concepts, and biology and physics, Einstein and Freud were approaching the possible convergence of the earliest mystics' claims that absolute knowledge is possible by activating the "subtle anatomy" and Reissner's fiber. Einstein and Freud did not travel that road. But by imagining an alternate history in which they did, we might better understand the psychological and conceptual barriers that have prevented progress along that road.

Freud's parents came from a Chasidic background, a branch of Judaism organized around the Kabbalah. He undoubtedly was familiar with the symbols of the *Sephirot* and its relationship with Absolute. However, Freud saw himself as a "conquistador" who, like Einstein, would seek truth along the road of science. Although Freud had initially aligned his scientific goal with the Manifesto's goal of bringing physics and psychology together, in 1895 he abandoned his *Project for a Scientific Psychology* which attempted "…to furnish a psychology that shall be a natural science; that is, to represent psychical processes as quantitatively determinate states of specifiable material particles, thus making the processes perspicuous and free from contradiction."

Freud was confused, torn, and tormented by his quest. To his colleague Wilhelm Fliess, an otolaryngologist, whose theory of neurosis based on sexual biorhythms linking genitalia with the nasal mucosa had impressed him, Freud wrote:

> My tyrant is psychology; it has always been my distant, beckoning goal, and now, since I have hit on the neuroses, … I am plagued with two

ambitions: to see how the theory of mental functioning takes shape if quantitative considerations, a sort of economics of nerve-force, are introduced into it; and secondly, to extract from psychopathology what may be of benefit to normal psychology.

Freud, outwardly, rejected the kabbalistic wellsprings understanding, knowledge, and wisdom. He also soon abandoned his *Project for a Scientific Psychology*. In 1895, shortly before abandoning it and hiding it in his desk drawer, Freud wrote to Fliess:

> During one industrious night last week the barriers suddenly lifted, the veils dropped and everything became transparent—from the details of the neuroses to the determinants of consciousness. Everything seemed to fall into place, the cogs meshed. I had the impression that the thing now really was a machine that shortly would function on its own.

But several weeks later, he wrote, "I no longer understand the state of mind in which I hatched the psychology; cannot conceive how I could have inflicted it on you. I believe you are still too polite; to me it appears to have been a kind of madness."

In 1895, in *Studies on Hysteria*, cowritten with Josef Breuer, whose cathartic talking cure of Anna O. inspired Freud's development of psychoanalysis, Freud wrote:

> In what follows little mention will be made of the brain and none whatever of molecules. Psychical processes will be dealt with in the language of psychology; and indeed, it cannot possibly be otherwise ... For while ideas are constant objects of our experience and are familiar to us in all their shades of meaning, "cortical excitations" are on the contrary rather in the nature of a postulate, objects which we hope to be able to identify in the future. The substitution of one term for another would seem to be no more than a pointless disguise.

Ultimately, he abandoned his *Project for a Scientific Psychology* as "premature" because "according to the view of our natural science, to which psychology must be subjected here, there are only masses in motion and nothing else." While lamenting that his new science of psychoanalysis was "floating in air," Freud followed what he called the "royal road to the unconscious," the "Holy Writ" of dreams. Reminiscent of his earlier exuberance about his *Project for a Scientific Psychology*, Freud wrote to Fliess, "Do you suppose that some day a marble tablet will be placed on the house, inscribed with these words: 'In this house on July 24th, 1895, the secret of dreams was revealed to Dr. Sigmund Freud?'"

As Freud struggled to find a material basis of psychology, his father tried to persuade him to find inspiration in the Kabbalah. In 1891, as Freud was struggling to develop a materialist psychology, his father

Is Science a Vestige of the Search for Lost Hallucinatory Gods? 113

put new leather binding on Sigmund's (ne Shlomoh's) Hebrew Bible and sent it to his son as a gift for his thirty-fifth birthday. Inscribed in the front, written in Hebrew, was a mosaic consisting of Biblical verses and other Jewish sources (sources added):

> Son who is dear to me, Shlomoh, [Jeremiah]
> In the seventh in the days of the years of your life [Genesis] the Spirit of the Lord began to move you [Judges]
> and spoke within you: Go, read in my Book that I have written [Exodus] and there will burst open for you the wellsprings of understanding, knowledge and wisdom.
> Behold, it is in the Book of Books, from which sages have excavated and lawmakers learned [Numbers, Judges] knowledge and justice.
> A vision of the Almighty did you see; [Numbers] you heard and strove to do, [Exodus]
> and you soared upon the wings of the Spirit.
> Since then the Book has been stored [Deuteronomy] like the fragments of the Tablets in an ark with me.
> For the day on which your years were filled to five and thirty
> I have put upon a cover of new skin [Numbers]
> and have called it: "Spring up, O well, sing ye unto it!" [Numbers] and I have presented it to you as a memorial [Exodus] and as a reminder.

Although Freud, in his later years, denied the ability to read Hebrew, his father's inscription was written in the original language of the Bible. Red, green, and blue colored pencils matching the underlinings of Hebrew passages in his Bible were discovered in Freud's desk drawer when he died. Freud's father's passionate plea, "Go read in my Book and there will burst open for you the wellsprings of understanding, knowledge and wisdom," is an explicit reference to the Kabbalah. Understanding, knowledge, and wisdom are the uppermost triad of the *Sephirot*—*binah*, *da'at*, and *chochma*—the spheres communicating God's will, our meaning and purpose. They are the acronym of Chabad, the largest Chasidic group in the world.

Although Freud suppressed and disguised his kabbalist roots, recently disclosed diary entries by Rabbi Shalom Dov-Ber Schneersohn —the 5th Lubavitcher Rebbe, the leader of Chabad—describe meetings with Freud in Vienna between 1902 and 1903. The following conversation reveals a tantalizing metaphor for Reissner's fiber.

> *Rebbe*: "The discipline of *Chassidut* requires that 'the head explains to the heart what the person should want, and that the heart implement in the person's life that which the head understands.'"

> *Freud*: "How do you do this? Are not the head and heart two continents completely separated? Does not a great sea divide them?"

Rebbe: "The task is to build a bridge that will span these two continents, or at least to connect them with telephone lines and electric wires so that the light of the mind, the light of the brain, should reach the heart as well."

Freud's well-known pathologizing of religion was based in large part on dissimulation to protect psychoanalysis from the virulent anti-Semitism in Vienna. He anointed Carl Jung as his heir and the guarantor that psychoanalysis would not become a "Jewish national affair."

Shortly before he signed the 1912 Manifesto, another opportunity to investigate the possibility that the earliest mystics' claims that absolute knowledge is possible by activating the "subtle anatomy" could be realized by Reissner's fiber presented itself. In 1912, Jung published his first work on *kundalini*, and Tantric and Taoist yoga, *Transformation and Symbols of the Libido*. However, in 1913, tensions between Freud and Jung led to a bitter split. Freud pleaded to Jung, "Promise me never to abandon the sexual theory—make a dogma of it, an unshakable bulwark against the black tide of mud of occultism." Jung accused Freud of "soulless materialism."

Freud stood poised to follow the 1912 Manifesto's inspiration to pursue a convergence of physics, biology, and psychology upon the Absolute by identifying the Reissner's fiber with the "subtle anatomy." But the Devil detoured that quest. Although Reissner's fiber's existence as a biological structure was well established, it had been cast out of the neuroscientific paradigm as an elastic cord. Freud further distanced himself from the fiber by abandoning his *Project for a Scientific Psychology* for his psychoanalytic castle floating in air.

In 1927, Einstein and Freud met for the only time. Afterward, Freud wrote to a friend about his meeting: "He understands as much about psychology as I do about physics, so we had a very pleasant talk." When a friend wrote Einstein just a few months after his meeting with Freud suggesting that he undergo psychoanalysis, he answered, "I should like very much to remain in the darkness of not having been analyzed." Regarding Freudian psychoanalysis Einstein once wrote, "His theories are lost on me because my personal life has no live material."

During the fifteen years that had passed between the signing of the 1912 Manifesto and their meeting, Freud had begun to break through some of the dissimulations and psychological defenses that had distanced him from his Chasidic heritage to search for the "telephone lines and electric wires" that could connect the heart and brain. In 1920, Rabbi Chayim Bloch had been asked by his mentor, the eminent Rabbi

Joseph Bloch, to do a German translation of the works of Chayim Vital, a sixteenth-century rabbi who had been the most important student of Isaac Luria, a great kabbalist who laid the foundation of our modern understanding of the relationship between the microcosm of man and the macrocosmic Adam Kadmon. Luria's teachings were delivered as impromptu lectures. Chayim Vital recorded all of them, eventually compiling them into many volumes.

Chayim Bloch, however, lost interest in the project soon after he had begun, and abandoned it altogether when Joseph Bloch died in 1923. Shortly thereafter, however, following a dream in which Joseph Bloch came to him and asked him why he had not finished the project, Chayim Bloch completed the translation.

Believing that Chayim Vital's work could contribute to our understanding of psychology, Chayim Bloch reached out to Freud and asked him to write a forward to the book and to help with its publication. Freud agreed and they met in Freud's library. After reading the manuscript, Freud exclaimed to Bloch, "This is gold!" and asked why Chayim Vital's work had never been brought to his attention in the past. Given Freud's passion to establish sexuality as the bedrock of psychology, his exultant reaction resulted from Lurianic Kabbalah's cosmic perspective on sexuality: sacred sexuality mirrors the union of the exiled feminine counterpart of God, *Shekinah*, and God.

Freud informed Bloch that he too had written a book that was relevant to Judaism, and showed him the manuscript of *Moses and Monotheism*. After skimming the pages, it quickly became apparent to Bloch that Freud had blamed the Jews for killing their greatest prophet and liberator. An argument ensued and Freud angrily left the room. Alone in Freud's library, Bloch browsed the shelves. To his dismay, he found a translation of the classical kabbalistic text, the *Zohar*, as well as several German books on Jewish mysticism.

In 1927, Freud received a letter from his friend, the mystic Romain Rolland, in response to reading the copy of *Future of an Illusion* he had sent him. Rolland replied that while he agreed that many followers of religion engage in superstitious, ritualistic behaviors based on illusions and deceptions of the clergy, the source and essence of religion is something deeper. Rolland believed that religion derives from a sensation of eternity, something limitless, oceanic. He believed that organized, institutionalized religion had misdirected this energy and ultimately depleted it. Contemplation of Rolland's ideas further lifted layers of suppressions and repressions of Freud's religious longings.

In 1929, when he was 73, Freud wrote in the beginning of his book, *Civilization and Its Discontents*:

> The views expressed by the friend whom I so much honor, and who himself once praised the magic of illusion in a poem caused me no small difficulty ... From my own experience I could not convince myself of the primary nature of such a feeling. But this gives me no right to deny that it does in fact occur in other people. The only question is whether it is being correctly interpreted and whether it ought to be regarded as the *fons et origo* of the whole need for religion.

In the preface to the Hebrew translation of *Totem and Taboo* written in 1930, Freud wrote:

> If the question were put to him: "Since you have abandoned all these common characteristics of your countrymen, what is there left to that is Jewish?" he would reply: "A very great deal, and probably its essence." He could not now express that essence clearly in words; but some day, no doubt, it will be accessible to the scientific mind.

In 1933, in his *New Introductory Lectures on Psychoanalysis*, Freud expressed a new openness toward mysticism. While expressing skepticism about "other worlds," paranormal phenomena, and miracles, he confessed that, "If one regards oneself as a skeptic, it is a good plan to have occasional doubts about one's skepticism too. It may be that I too have a secret inclination towards the miraculous which thus goes halfway to meet the creation of occult facts."

While some ludicrous ideas such as the hypothesis that "jam is at the center of the earth" should be immediately rejected, he wrote, it is "erroneous and detrimental" to immediately reject all ideas that do not conform to our current intellectual framework. Freud compared the initial condemnation of the hypothesized unconscious substratum of consciousness to the condemnation mystics have encountered throughout the ages.

In 1937, Freud, in *Moses and Monotheism*, wrote:

> There is an element of grandeur about everything to do with the origin of a religion, certainly including the Jewish one, and this is not matched by the explanations [I] have hitherto given. Some other factor must be involved to which there is little that is analogous and nothing that is of the same kind, something unique and something of the same order of magnitude as what has come out of it, religion itself.

As Freud neared death, he wrote to the chief rabbi of Vienna: "In some place in my soul, in a hidden corner, I am a fanatical Jew. I am very much astonished to discover myself as such in spite of all efforts to be unprejudiced and impartial."

When Freud met with Einstein, what he had perceived as the "black tide of mud of occultism" was becoming a receding tide that was revealing lost secrets. Somewhere in the depths of his unconscious, childhood images of the anatomy of Adam Kadmon were being reawakened along with the images of the "subtle anatomy" of *kundalini* and Taoist yoga that he had learned about from Jung. Their unmistakable resemblance to Reissner's fiber could not have gone unnoticed in Freud's freely associating unconscious mind. The tormented passion to ground consciousness in physics was silently calling out from the depths of his unconscious, calling out to the dreamer in his psychoanalytic castle floating in air.

What If?

What if, during their 1927 meeting, Einstein and Freud had revisited the 1912 Manifesto? Is absolute knowledge attainable? Indeed, is it conceivable? Einstein would have rejected the notion of absolute knowledge. For Einstein, we stand before "that what is impenetrable to us" with "rapturous amazement" and wonder without any legitimate way of going beyond.

Freud was beginning to re-examine man's relationship with the limitless, eternal essence of religion. Freud was beginning his scientific quest for the origin of religion.

Had Freud shared the transformation occurring in the hidden corners of his soul, Einstein might have shared the traumatic childhood experience that had convinced him that religion is a primitive superstition perpetuated by lying clergy. While Einstein preferred to remain in the darkness of not having been analyzed because his personal life had no live material, Freud might have repeated the admonition contained his just published *Future of an Illusion*:

> Truths contained in religious doctrines are, after all, so distorted and systematically disguised that the mass of humanity cannot recognize them as truth. The case is similar to what happens when we tell a child that new-born babies are brought by the stork. Here, too, we are telling the truth in symbolic clothing, for we know what the large bird signifies. But the child does not know it. He hears only the distorted part of what we say, and feels that he has been deceived; and we know how often his distrust of the grown-ups and his refractoriness actually take their start from this impression. We have become convinced that it is better to avoid such symbolic disguisings of the truth in what we tell children and not to withhold from them a knowledge of the true state of affairs commensurate with their intellectual level.

While Freud's words probably would not have changed Einstein's attitude, they might have led Freud back to his childhood Chasidic influences, to his father's cryptic Hebrew message inscribed on the front of a leather bound Bible, and to Jung's investigations of the symbols of yoga. Reissner's fiber, that had glimmered under his microscope in Brucke's lab, was swirling around repressed images of the "subtle anatomy."

Following the Manifesto's recognition that contemplation of the possibility of absolute knowledge leads directly to the question of the connection between thought and the brain and the relationship between physics and biology, Freud might have shared the story of his abandoned quest for a scientific psychology grounded in physics. Explaining that he had abandoned his project after realizing that physics, at the time, dealt only with masses in motion and nothing else, Einstein might have introduced Freud to the emerging controversy regarding the role of consciousness in quantum mechanics. In 1927, Einstein, the reluctant godfather of quantum mechanics, was seeing his unruly godchild being hailed as the revealer of the mystical underbelly of science. Mere matter in motion was transforming into an immaterial reality that resembled mind and spirit.

Pondering quantum mechanics' implication that very small things become insubstantial beyond the threshold of Planck's constant and that material reality isn't really there until it is observed, and following the Manifesto's roadmap toward the convergence of physics and biology upon psychology, the swirling, Freud's reawakened images of the "subtle anatomy" might have connected with Reissner's fiber. However, had Freud put the elusive, neglected enigmatic fiber on the table as the biological structure upon which physics and psychology converge, Einstein would have seen a problem. Reissner's fiber, a meter-long fiber immersed in the warm, wet, noisy CSF, could seemingly not exist as a quantum system. At the time, prior to theories of decoherence and multiverses, the designation of macroscopic systems as classical was based on the "Correspondence Principle," that Arnold Sommerfield, who supervised several Nobel Prize winners, had dubbed "Bohr's magic wand."

Scientists first glimpsed macroscopic quantum behaviors in 1908, when, after twenty-five years of frantic, intense effort, Heike Kamerlingh Onnes at the University of Leiden in the Netherlands first liquefied helium. As Onnes began investigating the properties of liquid helium, he discovered something remarkable: the electrical resistance plummeted to zero. He called this new phenomena superconductivity.

At first, Onnes embraced Einstein's idea of quantum oscillators that he had used explain specific heats to explain the drop in electrical resistance. But it soon became apparent that this explanation was inadequate. Einstein struggled to explain superconductivity. In 1922, he wrote:

> Given our ignorance of quantum mechanics of composite systems we are far away from being able to convert these vague ideas into a theory ... Fantasizing can only be excused by the momentary quandary of the theory. It is obvious that new ways of serving the facts have to be found.

In 1924, Satyendra Nath Bose developed a novel way to derive quantum statistics based on the idea that photons and other similar particles can be conceptualized as indistinguishable particles now known as bosons. Bose, an unknown physicist, sent his paper to Einstein, who immediately recognized its significance, translated it himself, and sent it out for publication in a prestigious journal. That same year, Einstein proposed that below a certain temperature quantum system could from macroscopic, coherent quantum systems now known as Bose-Einstein condensations. On November 29, 1924, Einstein sent a letter to his friend Paul Ehrenfest: "From a certain temperature on, the molecules 'condense' without attractive forces, that is, they accumulate at zero velocity. The theory is pretty, but is there also some truth in it?" At the time, most physicists regarded Einstein's speculation as imaginary.

In 1924, Onnes observed another remarkable property of liquid helium: it undergoes a phase transition in which its density spikes. Little attention was paid to these remarkable results until 1938, when Pyotr Kapitza observed that liquid helium has zero viscosity. Analogizing his discovery with superconductors, he called this new state of matter a superfluid. That same year, Fritz London proposed that Bose-Einstein condensations could explain superfluidity and superconductivity. Controversy and confusion amidst competing explanations ensued. It continues to this day. There are clearly other factors involved in the phenomenon of superfluidity and other macroscopic phenomena than Bose-Einstein condensation. It was not until 1995 that the first actual Bose-Einstein condensations were produced in a gas of rubidium atoms cooled to near absolute zero. Subsequently other atoms, molecules, and photons were cooled to create Bose-Einstein condensations.

Cooling to temperatures near absolute zero would not be a suitable method of transforming Reissner's fiber into a macroscopic quantum system in a living brain. However, Einstein had begun to ponder other mechanisms that might produce macroscopic quantum systems. In 1917, Einstein presented a paper on the quantization of energy in quantum systems that would lead to a new understanding. This paper, titled "On the Quantum Theorem of Sommerfeld and Epstein," showed the limits of the old quantum mechanics when applied to chaotic systems. It was ignored for twenty-five years and it was not until 1973 that Ian Percival reintroduced the connection between Einstein's insights and quantum chaos to the physics community. Gabor Vatay proposed the possibility that quantum chaos might produce macroscopic, biological quantum coherences in 2012.

But even if Einstein had envisioned Reissner's fiber as a macroscopic quantum system, he would have confronted contradictions in his philosophical stance regarding the relationship between mind and matter. On the one hand, the postulation of a physical reality that exists independent of consciousness was the foundation of his scientific philosophy and he reconciled himself to the commission of the metaphysical original sin. On the other hand, he had asserted, "I am fascinated by Spinoza's pantheism, but I admire even more his contribution to modern thought because he is the first philosopher to deal with the soul and body as one, and not two separate things." Spinoza resolved the apparent duality between body and soul by proposing that we have adequate knowledge of our body only when we known it "under a form of eternity," a realm beyond space and time. Reissner's fiber as a macroscopic quantum system is measurable as an object that moves through space and time. However, the zero point field surrounding it and occupying its hollow core is not.

The idea of zero point fluctuations was introduced in 1912 by Max Planck to explain discontinuous emission of radiation. In 1913, Einstein tried to calculate the specific heat of hydrogen gas on the basis of zero point fluctuations but soon retracted the idea, declaring in a letter to Paul Ehrenfest that the idea is "dead as doornail." However, in 1920, Einstein concluded that general relativity is inconceivable without the zero point energy of empty space. In 1927, Dirac provided a mathematical and conceptual basis for the zero point fluctuations of the physical vacuum; the creation and annihilation of virtual particles and antiparticles. A mathematical and conceptual model of the physical vacuum's interaction with a non-equilibrium macroscopic quantum system lies beyond our current understanding.

The road not traveled by Einstein and Freud (or traveled in a parallel universe according to the many-worlds interpretation of quantum mechanics), leads to a unified neurocosmology organized around Reissner's fiber. It is a road from the beginning of the past to the end of the future, beyond the "stubbornly persistent illusion" separating past, present, and future, to the place where physics, biology, psychology, anthropology, and history converge upon the Absolute.

Conclusion

Jaynes's notion that science is nostalgia for the lost certainty of hallucinatory gods and that scientific understanding is the feeling of familiarity with concrete metaphors is false. Einstein's epistemology based on free creations of thought and mathematics has been verified by empirical facts. It evokes cosmic religious feelings because of its revelations of natural laws that reflect a superior intelligence.

But Einstein's scientific road to God's thoughts is founded on a the metaphysical original sin. Can we atone? According to Einstein, the metaphysical original sin is necessary to avoid solipsism. Berkeley avoided this consequence of Idealistic philosophy by postulating that God is the ultimate perceiver whose perceptions give physical reality its legitimacy.

Einstein's scientific road to God's thoughts stopped short of knowing Him like the prophets, saints, and mystics have claimed lest he become a "victim of the clergy." He also stopped short of knowing God knowing the body under a form of eternity as Spinoza proposed. He also avoided the implications of Schrödinger's axioms—"I am God almighty"—by denying free will. However, this denial contradicts the foundation of his epistemology, free creations of thought.

By following Einstein's journey from his childhood religious paradise to his scientific paradise and Spinoza's God we find repressed, disguised, and ignored ideas from the Kabbalah and neuroscience. Wary of becoming victims of the "clergy," we can scientifically explore the realm beyond the limits of mathematics and physics by developing a unified neurocosmology organized around Reissner's fiber.

Six

Reissner's Fiber, the "Subtle Anatomy," and the Devil

According to yogic tradition, the first yogi, the Adiyoga, transmitted the secrets of the "subtle anatomy" to the first seven *rishis* more that 6,000 years ago. The Yellow Emperor of China, who is said to have reigned from 2698 to 2598 BC codified the esoteric teachings of the flow if *Qi* through the meridians and vessels. According to the Kabbalah, on September 7, 3761 BC the secrets of the *Sephirot,* the anatomy of Adam Kadmon, the Primordial Anthropos, the divine image in which man was created, the Tree of Life, were revealed to Adam and engraved in sapphire by the angel Raziel as *The Book of Raziel.* Ever since, Lailah, the Angel of Conception, places a lighted candle at the head of each unborn infant as it grows in the womb so that it sees the universe from its beginning to its end. She teaches the unborn the secrets of the eternal blueprint of creation. As the baby emerges from the womb, Lailah lightly strikes the newborn above the lip causing him to forget all her teachings. Lailah watches over him as the silent voice of God.

Reissner's Fiber and the Central Pillar of the *Sephirot*

Revelations from angels purportedly encrypted in the esoteric layers of the Old Testament would seem to be unworthy of serious scientific consideration. Creationism, based on a literal interpretation of Genesis, is scientifically ridiculous. The notion that our earliest ancestors knew about cosmological and neuropsychological phenomena that are just now becoming accessible to modern science appears to be preposterous. However, the hypothesis that the Kabbalah originated from interoceptions of Reissner's fiber creates a new perspective. The fetal involution of the fiber is echoed by the story of Lailah.

Just beneath the surface of the literal meaning of the Torah is an interpretation that is in accord with modern cosmology. The *Sefer*

HaTemunah, an early kabbalistic work attributed to the first-century rabbinic sage Tanna Nehunya ben ha-Kanah that analyzes the significance of the geometry of Hebrew letters also proposed that the universe underwent six, 7,000-year-long Sabbatical cycles before Adam and therefore calculated that the universe is 42,000 years old. In the thirteenth century, Rabbi Isaac of Akko wrote, "I, the insignificant Yitzchak of Akko, have seen fit to write a great mystery that should be kept very well hidden. One of God's days is a thousand years, as it says, 'For a thousand years are in Your eyes as a fleeting yesterday.' Since one of our years is 365 ¼ days, a year on High is 365,250 of our years. For a thousand years in thy sight are but like yesterday when it is past, and like a watch in the night" (Psalms 90:4). 42,000 multiplied by 365,250 is 15,340,500,000. Current estimates of the age of the universe are 13.82 billion, but uncertainties introduced by dark matter and relativistic effects during the very early universe might raise the current estimate.

As Robert Jastrow wrote in *God and the Astronomers*:

> For the scientist who has lived by his faith in the power of reason, the story ends like a bad dream. He has scaled the mountains of ignorance, he is about to conquer the highest peak; as he pulls himself over the final rock, he is greeted by a band of theologians who have been sitting there for centuries.

But there is much more than mere agreement between theologians and cosmologists that the universe had a beginning. The cosmological constant, Einstein's "blunder" that was revived after the expansion of the universe was observed to be accelerating, is so finely tuned that if the value of the trillionth, trillionth, trillionth, trillionth, trillionth, trillionth, trillionth, trillionth, trillionth, trillionth decimal point were different, the universe would have expanded so fast that there would have been no galaxies or stars. The improbability of the order of that initial singularity is so great that a number generated by placing a "0" on every particle in the universe would be vanishingly small compared to it. According to the Anthropic Principle of cosmology, the remarkable fine-tuning of the physical constants implies that the universe was designed for sentient observers.

The theological implications of the Anthropic Principle and the contemplation of the question of how something came from nothing have softened the atheistic implications of Darwinism. For those imbued with the belief that science is waging a battle against blind faith, superstition, and the supernatural, there is an uneasy feeling that science's abandonment of Newton's search for the *prisca sapientia* was premature. Such feelings were expressed by Professor of Astronomy George Greenstein:

> It was not for some time that I was able to place my finger on the source of my discomfort. It arises, I understand now, because the contention that we owe our existence to a stupendous series of coincidences strikes a responsive chord. That contention is far too close for comfort to notions such as: We are the center of the universe. God loves mankind more than all other creatures. The cosmos is watching over us. The universe has a plan; we are essential to that plan.

For Leonard Susskind, author of *The Cosmic Landscape: String Theory and the Illusion of Intelligent Design*, the discomforting theological implications of the Anthropic Prinicple must be combated at all costs:

> Maybe God did make the world. But scientists—real scientists—resist the temptation to explain natural phenomena, including creation itself, by divine intervention. Why? Because as scientists we understand that there is a compelling need to believe—the need to be comforted—that easily clouds people's judgement. It's all too easy to fall into the seductive trap of a comforting fairy tale. So, we resist to the death, all explanations of the world based on anything but the Laws of Physics, mathematics and probability.

Susskind's battle to the death against divine intervention compels him to embrace the theory of cosmic landscapes. According to this theory, the nothingness from which the universe was created, the physical vacuum, existed as a nearly infinite (10^{500}) array of vacua. Each of these vacua spawned inflating bubble universes that exist beyond our cosmic horizon. The "stupendous series of coincidences" that we observe in our universe is a result of a lucky accident.

While contemplation of the implications of modern cosmology has converted some scientists to deism, few scientists, especially biologists, are theists. The idea of a God who directed organic evolution and who interacts with the volitional activity of humans contravenes evolutionary and neuroscientific orthodoxy. Following Darwinism's defeat of Creationism, Thomas Huxley, "Darwin's bulldog," famously wrote:

> Extinguished theologians lie about the cradle of science as the strangled snakes beside that of Hercules; and history records that whenever science and orthodoxy have been fairly opposed, the latter has been forced to retire from the lists, bleeding and crushed, if not annihilated, scotched if not slain.

But, as the molecular level of life was uncovered during the twentieth century, theologians who searched beyond the literal interpretation of Genesis joined with scientists to question the proposition that random variation and natural selection alone were sufficient ot explain the origin of life and the evolution from bacteria to man. It comes down to a question of calculating probabilities.

Darwin believed that variations are not due to chance:

> I have hitherto sometimes spoken as if the variations—so common and multiform in organic beings under domestication, and in a lesser degree in those in a state of nature—had been due to chance. This, of course, is a wholly incorrect expression, but it serves to acknowledge plainly our ignorance of the cause of each particular variation.

Furthermore, he believed "that the impossibility of conceiving that this grand and wondrous universe, with our conscious selves, arose through chance seems to me the chief argument for the existence of God." However, this argument was not sufficient to dissuade him from agnosticism. "I feel most deeply," he wrote, "that the whole subject is too profound for the human intellect. A dog might as well speculate on the mind of Newton. — Let each man hope & believe what he can."

It is unclear whether Darwin's belief that it is impossible to conceive that "this grand and wondrous universe, with our conscious selves, arose through chance" is a failure of imagination or a product of valid statistical analysis. The jury is still out.

Lost in the debate whether our conscious selves arose through chance or through unknown natural laws is the question whether consciousness arose from nonconscious matter at all. In 1859, Darwin concluded his *On the Origin of Species* with a lyrical depiction of life evolving from its "simple" beginning:

> There is grandeur in this view of life, with its several powers, having been originally breathed into a few forms or into one; and that, whilst this planet has gone cycling on according to the fixed law of gravity, from so simple a beginning endless forms most beautiful and most wonderful have been, and are being, evolved.

However, the following year, succumbing to pressure from those whose religious sensibilities were offended, Darwin expanded the phrase "having been originally breathed into a few forms or one," into "breathed *by the Creator* into a few forms or one." He soon regretted this decision. In 1863, he wrote to his closest friend, the distinguished botanist, Joseph Hooker:

> I have long regretted that I truckled to public opinion & used Pentateuchal term of creation, by which I really meant "appeared" by some wholly unknown process. It is mere rubbish thinking, at present, of origin of life; one might as well think of origin of matter.

One hundred fifty years later, with a deeper understanding of the initial singularity and the discovery of the Higgs boson, thinking about the origin of matter is no longer merely rubbish thinking. While Wallace's call for a "metaphysical imposition" to explain the origin of life and consciousness has been deemed to lie outside the boundaries of natural science, hyperspatial branes in a cosmic landscape of multiverse embraced by a hierarchy of infinities blur the boundaries between physics and metaphysics, between naturalism and supernaturalism. Our "simple" cosmic origins aren't so simple. The possibility of supersensory perceptions opens another door to the "supernatural."

The Kabbalistic "Subtle Anatomy" and the Devil

Reissner's fiber as an observable object has played its role as the Devil according Baudelaire for 150 years by concealing itself beneath layer of skin, muscle, bone, membranes, and neural tissue, disintegrating shortly after death, typically involuting perinatally in human, and operating with mechanisms that lie outside the neuroscientific paradigm. Reissner's fiber as a possible interoception described as by kabalists as the *Sephirot* is buried beneath the dust of fallen Babel, disguised, distorted, and fragmented.

According to the kabbalistic interpretation of Genesis, in the seventh generation after Adam, Enoch received the secrets revealed to Adam. He was the first to have internalized them. Genesis 5:24 succinctly says, "Enoch walked faithfully with God; then he was no more, because God took him away." He and Elijah are the only two individuals who are said to have ascended to heaven without dying. But, before God took Enoch, he passed the secrets to his great-grandson, Noah, who passed the secrets to Abraham. The secrets were transmitted from Abraham to Isaac, to Jacob and to Joseph, and then buried with his bones in a casket along the Nile River. Fulfilling a solemn pledge made by Joseph's brothers (Genesis 50:25), Moses retrieved the bones of Joseph and the secrets of *The Book of Raziel* on his way to free the Israelites from Egypt. By now, the oral secrets pertaining to the interoceptions of Reissner's fiber were 2,000 years old.

In the summer of 1313 BC, amidst thunder, lightning, smoke, and tremors, during the only collective revelation in human history, Moses ascended Mt. Sinai and received the written Torah, the blueprint of creation, and the secrets of integrating the vertical dimensions of the secrets transmitted from Eden with the horizontal dimensions of history. In the Five Books of Moses that have come down to us, one chapter is devoted to the creation of the universe. Thirteen chapters are devoted to the construction of a structure, the Tabernacle and the Ark of the Covenant that can contain the creator. The miracle of containing the infinite within a finite structure is far greater than the miracle of creating a finite world from the infinite.

That the blueprint for the Tabernacle and the Ark metaphorically refer to human anatomy is suggested by the verse, "And let them make me a sanctuary, that I may dwell in their midst" (Exodus 25:8). Rabbi Isaiah Horowitz (1558–1628), known as the Shaloh, explains that the verse does not say that God will dwell "in its midst" because it is referring to the sanctuary within each one of us. That the Ark also metaphorically refers to innermost spiritual dimensions of man is suggested by a Talmudic tale about measuring the Ark within the Holy of Holies in the First Temple in Jerusalem. The chamber of the Holy of Holies measured twenty cubits by twenty cubits and the ark measured two and a half by one and a half cubits. The Ark occupied the center of the chamber. The measurement from the southern wall of the chamber to the adjacent side of the ark was ten cubits. The same measurement was taken on the north side of the chamber. The Ark occupied no space!

The Kabbalah explains the intersection of the vertical and horizontal dimension of the Torah in terms of four levels of interpretation, that correspond to four planes of reality that relate to five levels of the soul. The first level of interpretation, *pshat*, is the explicit meaning, such as the historical facts. Next is *remez*, which finds hints of deeper meanings using methods such a gematria. Beneath *remez* is *derash*, which deals with the metaphorical and allegorical levels of meaning. Deeper meanings are also found by analyzing repetitions and phrasings. The deepest level is the secret, mystical level, *sod*. Here, the ontological and epistemological status of language goes beyond ordinary cognitive levels. There is an intrinsic connection between the geometry of the written letters and the vibrations of the spoken language words, the four planes of reality, and the five levels of the soul.

Moses taught the secrets of the intersection of the vertical and horizontal dimensions of the Torah to his brother Aaron and to the Elders. The physical embodiment of that intersection, the Tabernacle and Ark of the Covenant, constructed according to the specification revealed to Moses, was, after years of wandering the desert, brought to the tent of King David and then placed inside the King Solomon's Temple in Jerusalem in the mid-tenth century BC. The physical embodiments of the secrets were lost when the Babylonians destroyed the Temple in 586 BC. The reference to the *Sephirot*, the image of God in which man was created, is alluded to only in what appears to be a contradictory second story of creation in Genesis 2, which describes one day of creation during which *Elohim* created man and breathed life into him.

Following the Babylonian exile, and the end of prophecy, it was forbidden to commit the Oral Law to writing. Its deepest mystical secrets were transmitted to only one carefully selected and trained student at a time. According to one Talmudic commentary, only the Head of the supreme Rabbinical Court, if he were sufficiently wary, could receive the mystical teachings. These closely guarded teachings were called the *Ma'aseh Merkavah*, the "Work of the Chariot," based on Ezekiel's visions from the seventh century BC.

Jesus was undoubtedly familiar with the teachings of the Heads of supreme Rabbinical Court, Rabbis Hillel and Shammai. Jesus also proclaimed that the exoteric template of the mystical secrets of the Oral Law was sacred and the guide to his mission: "Do not think that I came to abolish the Law or the Prophets; I did not come to abolish but to fulfill. For truly I say to you, until heaven and earth pass away, not the smallest letter or stroke (one iota or one tittle) shall pass from the Law (Torah) until all is accomplished" (Matthew 5:18). While John's proclamation, "The Word became flesh and made his dwelling among us" (John 1:14), does not describe Jesus's specific anatomical connection with the "Word," there are stories from the Gospels and mysteries surrounding the Shroud of Turin that might shed light on the possible role of Reissner's fiber.

The Transfiguration described in the synoptic gospels (Matthew 17:1-8, Mark 9:2-8, Luke 9:28-36) tells of a meeting of Moses, Elijah, and Jesus. These are the only three men in the Bible who are said to have undergone fasts of 40 days and 40 nights. Matthew 17:2 states that Jesus "was transfigured before them; his face shining as the sun, and his garments became white as the light."

The miraculous defiance of dehydration, hypovolemic shock, and heat stroke might be evidence of their functioning Reissner's fibers. Reissner's fiber's two primary connections to the brain, the preoptic region of the hypothalamus and the subcommissural organ, regulate the hormones vasopressin, a water conserving, anti-diuretic, and aldosterone, a blood pressure elevator, respectively. The preoptic region of the hypothalamus is the brain's thermoregulatory center. The ending of Reissner's fiber in the terminal ventricle is surrounded by clusters of hormone secreting cells that were first identified in the terminal ventricle of fish. This hormone, urotensin II, which resembles rhodopsin, the photosensitive molecule in the retina, and which has been evolutionarily conserved for 560 million years, has been identified in humans as the most potent human vasoconstrictor. Reissner's fiber could have orchestrated the hormonal response that conserved water and maintained blood pressure. Reissner's fiber is connected with the brain's two key biological clocks, the preoptic region of hypothalamus and the pineal gland. Acting as the central controller of the biological clock, the fiber could have slowed metabolism, creating a state of suspended animation.

The image on the Shroud of Turin, the alleged burial shroud of Jesus, continues to baffle scientists. Philip Ball, who was the physical science editor of *Nature* when the journal published the carbon dating results that seemed to disprove the authenticity of the Shroud, wrote the following after credible new analysis opened the possibility that the Shroud is 2,000 years old:

> The scientific study of the Turin Shroud is like a microcosm of the scientific search for God. It does more to inflame any debate than settle it ... And yet, the shroud is a remarkable artifact, one of the few religious relics to have a justifiably mythical status. It is simply not known how the ghostly image of a serene, bearded man was made.

According to a theory proposed by Frank Tipler, professor of physics at Tulane University, the image on the Shroud was formed by neutrinos released from an obscure process involving "sphaleron baryon annihilation" produced by astronomically improbable quantum coherences. The creation of a burst of radiation from quantum coherences of Reissner's fiber would not require an astronomically improbable chance development if quantum coherences in the trillions of cells of the body, but rather the effects of quantum feedback and control by the circumventricular system.

While the accounts of mystical experiences occurring in the context of forty days of going without food or water in the Judean desert, and the image on the Shroud suggest the hypothesis that Reissner's fiber was present in Moses, Elijah, or Jesus, there are no writings in the Gospels about the anatomy of Adam Kadmon or the *Sephirot*.

About the time the first Gospels were being written, after the destruction of the second temple in Jerusalem in 70 AD, Rabbi Shimon Bar Yochai, a disciple of the leading kabbalist, Rabi Akiva, fled Roman persecution with his son to a cave. There, during a twelve-year period, inspired by the prophet Elijah, he wrote the foundational document of Kabbalah, the *Zohar*. Rabbinic edicts forbade pubic study of the mystical teachings. Subsequently, esoteric teachings related to the "subtle anatomy" were eclipsed by exoteric practices, the *mitzvoth*, the 613 commandments of the Torah.

The Kabbalah, as it has now come to be known, emerged during the thirteenth century when Rabbi Moses de Leon, a Spanish kabbalist, published the *Zohar*, claiming it to be a transcription of Rabbi Shimon Bar Yochai's original. During the sixteenth century, a group of kabbalists proclaiming divine inspiration, most notably Moshe Cordovero and later Isaac Luria, established schools in Safed, the highest city in the Galilee and Israel.

Cordovero systematized and developed kabbalistic thought. After his death in 1570, Luria presented a radically new understanding of Kabbalah that stressed the interaction between man and God to achieve universal redemption. Luria delivered his teachings as impromptu lectures. Only an elite group of initiates was taught the Kabbalah's esoteric secrets. Luria's most important initiate was Chayim Vital. His notes were compiled into numerous written works, the most important being the eight volume work, *The Tree of Life*. Copies of Vital's manuscripts were circulated among Luria's disciples who pledged never to take them from Israel to a foreign country. However, 200 years after Luria's death, in 1772, a copy was published in the Ukraine. By then Luria's teachings had spawned a variety of abstruse metaphysical interpretations.

Luria explained that the finite human world arose from an act of contraction of God's infinitude, *Tzimtzum*. A thin ray, *kav*, of God's infinite light, *Ohr-Ein-Sof*, emanated into the metaphysical void, *Tehiru*, created by *Tzimtzum*, and formed the *Sephirot* that constitute the body of Adam Kadmon. The vessels of the *Sephirot* shattered. Humankind's purpose is to elevate the "holy sparks" from the shattering of the vessels, *Shevirat Haelim*, to repair the world, *Tikkun ha-Olam*.

Luria, like all mystics, sought a way to know what is intellectually unknowable. Such knowing is embodied and lived. Physiology and cosmology are united. Guiding Luria's development of correspondences between the body and the cosmos was the anatomy of Adam Kadmon represented by the *Sephirot*. The chief problem for Luria was that Adam Kadmon exists in higher planes of reality beyond space and time. The correspondence between *kav*, the central axis of Adam Kadmon's anatomy and a one-dimensional quantum coherent thread ensheathed by Reissner's fiber was 350 years away.

Luria, therefore, used anatomical metaphors to bridge the gap between human anatomy and the anatomy of Adam Kadmon. Feet, limbs, and genitalia represented the lower *Sephirot*. The heart and brain represented the higher *Sephirot*. He also used explicit sexual terminology related to semen and vaginal fluids to represent the correspondences between the spiritual eroticism between man and wife and the conjugal flow between the masculine and feminine aspects of God. Because Luria's kabbalistic theosophy was an explication of the esoteric depths of the Torah, he also taught that the 248 "limbs" or "organs" and the 365 "tendons" or "veins" of Adam Kadmon correspond to the 248 negative and 365 positive commandments in the Torah and to the 248 organs and 365 tendons of human anatomy enumerated by Talmudic sages.

Following a decline in kabbalistic influence on Judaism, Rabbi Yisrael Baal Shem Tov, the founder of Chasidism, revived it and transformed its development during the nineteenth century. Opposing Chasidism were the followers of Rabbi Elijah ben Shlomo Zalman, commonly known as the Vilna Gaon. The Sages of Shklov, allies of the Vilna Gaon, interpreted the Zohar's proclamation, "And in the 600th year of the 6th millenium, (1840) the gates of upper wisdom will open, as well as the springs of lower wisdom, and the world will be repaired ahead of the 7th millennium," as a call for a synthesis of the esoteric depths of the Kabbalah with science. The seamless unity between spiritual and material reality that was cleaved with the first bite from the fruit of the Tree of Knowledge would be restored.

Eventually, Chasidism's charismatic leaders and its embrace of openness, tolerance, and joyful devotion to God attracted a large following. Chasidism became the voice of the Kabbalah. To safeguard kabbalism from idolatrous corporeal conceptions of God, it focused on spiritual and psychological interpretations of the *Sephirot*. According to Chasidic philosophy, science is subordinate to the Bible when apparent conflicts arise. Enthusiasm for a synthesis between Kabbalah and science as envisioned by the Sages of Shklov waned. But the esoteric teachings of the Kabbalah, closely guarded for millennia, would now be open to all.

The modern academic study of Kabbalah began with the pioneering work of Gershon Scholem during the mid twentieth century. However, he believed the symbols of Kabbalah were impenetrable. The writings of the Kabbalah were not primal revelations, but responses to historical crises of the Jewish people. While Scholem's influence continues to dominate the academic study of Kabbalah, other scholars, most notably Joseph Dan and Moshe Idel, have begun peeling away historical layers in search of Kabbalah's mystical roots. In 1978, Charles Ponce proposed that the *Sephirot* represent a "subtle anatomy" equivalent to the *nadis* and *chakras* of yoga. The first published proposal that the *Sushumna nadi* and the central pillar of the *Sephirot* are Reissner's fiber appeared in my 2016 article, "Reissner's Fibre: A Forgotten Pathway for Exploring Consciousness," in the *Journal of Consciousness Studies*.

For more than 5,000 years, infants have pre-consciously recapitulated the Biblical Fall. Ancient numinous visions, interoceptions of

Reissner's fiber, have called out to us from the depths of the personal and collective unconscious. Ancient texts, whose Hebrew letters once reflected the hyperspatial depths of reality and resonated with its higher vibrations, have appeared as fanciful, primitive myths and legends. But in the 600th year of the 6th millennium, the thread dangling free from the *Sephirot* began descending from the gates of upper wisdom toward Reissner's fiber rising from the springs of lower wisdom. The 1912 Manifesto provided a roadmap for Einstein and Freud to actualize the lost anatomical and cosmic secrets of the *Sephirot* into a neurocosmology organized around Reissner's fiber, but the Devil had other plans.

Yogic Subtle Anatomy

The *Sutras* of Pantajali written between the fifth and second century BC, depending on one's opinion regarding the scholarly evidence, are the first written record of the oral transmission of the Vedic secrets of the "subtle anatomy." It did little to inspire a search for a possible correspondence with physical human anatomy. And, human dissection was forbidden.

One of the earliest impetuses to investigate a possible biological basis of the "subtle anatomy" came from Swami Vivekananda, a disciple of the Indian mystic Ramakrishna. He had gained fame in the United States when he delivered speech to the Parliament of the World's Religions on September 11, 1893 where he was hailed by American newspapers as "the greatest figure in the parliament of religions" and "the most popular and influential man in the parliament." When some at the Parliament had questioned Vivekananda about his credentials, Harvard professor John Henry Wright exclaimed, "To ask for your credentials is like asking the sun to state its right to shine in the heavens."

In 1895, after Reissner's fiber's existence had been denied by leading anatomists for thirty-five years, Swami Vivekananda delivered a speech in London, where he explained *kundalini* as follows:

> According to the Yogis there are two nerve currents in the spinal column, called Pingalâ and Idâ, and a hollow canal called Sushumna running through the spinal cord. At the lower end of the hollow canal is what the Yogis call the "Lotus of the Kundalini". They describe it as triangular in form in which, in the symbolical language of the Yogis, there is a power called the Kundalini, coiled up. When that Kundalini awakes, it tries to force a passage through this hollow canal, and as it rises step by step, as it were, layer after layer of the mind becomes open and all the different visions and wonderful powers come to the Yogi. When it reaches the brain, the Yogi is perfectly detached from the body

and mind; the soul finds itself free. We know that the spinal cord is composed in a peculiar manner. If we take the figure eight horizontally (∞) there are two parts which are connected in the middle. Suppose you add eight after eight, piled one on top of the other, that will represent the spinal cord. The left is the Ida, the right Pingala, and that hollow canal which runs through the centre of the spinal cord is the Sushumna. Where the spinal cord ends in some of the lumbar vertebrae, a fine fibre issues downwards, and the canal runs up even within that fibre, only much finer.

Vivekananda's description of the *Sushumna nadi* as a hollow canal running through the spinal cord corresponds precisely to the central canal. The triangular "Lotus of the Kundalini" at the lower end of the central canal, within which the *kundalini* coils, corresponds to the triangular-shaped dilation at the end of the central canal called the terminal ventricle, within which Reissner's fiber coils. The fine fiber that issues forth from the end of the spinal cord corresponds to the delicate strand known as the filum terminale. "[T]he canal that runs up even within that fibre, only much finer," is the hollow tube which runs through the center of Reissner's fiber which runs upward from the filum terminal, to the terminal ventricle and up through the central canal.

However, in 1895, neuroscientists were disputing Reissner's fiber's existence as an actual biological structure. It did not appear in textbooks. It is very unlikely, therefore, that Vivekananda was aware if it.

Vivekananda's failure to identify Reissner's fiber as the conductor of *kundalini* within the central canal is, therefore, unsurprising. However, his conclusion that the "Lotus of the Kundalini," also known as the *Mooladara chakra*, corresponds to the sacral plexus, and that the "lotuses" or *chakras* correspond to plexuses that have their centers in the spinal canal, is puzzling. It is inconsistent with yogic texts and neuroanatomy. First, yogis describe the "Lotus of the Kundalini" as being directly below and continuous with the *Sushumna nadi*. The sacral plexus is several inches away from the end of the spinal cord, outside the sacral vertebrae. Second, the plexuses do not have their centers within the spinal canal. They lie outside the spinal canal, which is formed by the vertebrae. Third, the "lotuses" or *chakras* are described as being aligned with the *Sushumna nadi*, the central canal of the spinal cord, while nerve plexuses wander asymmetrically throughout the body. Fourth, Vivekananda makes unsupportable assertions regarding the probable mechanism by which the *kundalini* ascends from the *Mooladara chakra* to the *Sasarara chakra* in the brain. He claims that coiling of the *kundalini* in the *Mooladara chakra* refers to a heating up of energy, comparable to electricity, that can be consciously directed to ascend through the *Sushumna nadi* to attain "Divine Wisdom, superconscious perception, realisation of the spirit." However, neural signals from the sacral plexus do not travel to the terminal ventricle or central canal. They travel along neural pathways ascending the anterior and posterior tracts of the spinal cord carrying sensory input and motor output to the thighs, lower leg, foot, and part of the pelvis. Nevertheless, owing in large part to Vivekananda's fame and influence, his proposal has dominated subsequent searches for the anatomical basis of yoga.

In 1899, the same year that Porter Sargent became aware of the astonishing neglect of the peculiar, conspicuous, strategically located, evolutionarily persistent fiber, Sir John Woodroffe, an Oxford educated lawyer, traveled to British India where he became Supreme Justice of the Calcutta High Court and Tagore Law Professor at Calcutta University. Under the pseudonym Arthur Avalon (a play on King Arthur's mystical adventures on the island of Avalon chosen to convey his desire to link Western esotericism with lost mystical secrets of India), Woodroffe translated several ancient texts from their original Sanskrit, lectured and wrote extensively about Tantric philosophy, and played a prominent role in popularizing and stimulating academic interest in Hindu philosophy and yoga in the West. His book *Serpent Power*, a detailed description and explanation of the practices of Tantric yoga and the anatomical basis of *kundalini* yoga, based on his translation of *Shatchakra Nirupana* ("Description of and Investigation into the Six Bodily Centres") and the *Paduka-Panhcaka* ("Five-fold Footstool of the Guru"), first published in 1918, is still in print. He also wrote essays and commentaries trying to defend Tantric yoga against vociferous critics who denounced it as irrational, obscurantist, and prurient.

Woodroffe refined Vivekananda's diverted identification of the *Sushumna nadi* with the central canal. Having located the *Vajra nadi* within the *Sushumna nadi*, Woodroffe translated the second verse of the *Shatchakra Nirupana* as "Inside the *Vajra* is *Chittra* … She is subtle as a spider's thread." Inside the *Chittra nadi* is the innermost *nadi*, the *Brahma nadi*. The *Brahma-randhra*, the entrance to the *Brahma nadi*, is according to Woodroffe's translation of the forty-eighth verse "extremely subtle and like unto the ten-millionth part of the end of a hair."

Woodroffe's descriptions of the innermost *nadis* provided an accurate roadmap to Reissner's fiber. And, Woodroffe was likely one of the few people in the world who knew of the fiber. Ironically, the source of this knowledge was likely the person who helped the Devil push the fiber back to the backwaters of science after it had been briefly brought into the spotlight by Sargent, George Nicholls. In 1912, the year that Einstein and Freud had signed the Manifesto declaring the search for the absolute knowledge and the convergence of physics, biology, and psychology, as Woodroffe was completing one of his first works on Tantric yoga, Nicholls came to Calcutta on an academic assignment as he was completing his first investigations of Reissner's fiber. His characterization of the fiber as an elastic cord that ended in a "terminal plug" had allowed the fiber to play its role as the Devil according to Baudelaire. However, assuming that Woodroffe and Nicholls met for tea, presumably the latter told the former of his work on the now obscure fiber.

However, Woodroffe would not be the first to document the identification of Reissner's fiber with the central pathway of the *kundalini*. In 1927, Vasant Rele, a student of Woodroffe, who likely learned of the fiber from him, wrote the following glossary entry defining the *Vajra nadi* for his book *Mysterious Kundalini: The Physical Basis of the "kundali (Hatha) Yoga" in Terms of Western Anatomy and Physiology*: "A nerve fibre said to exist inside the spinal canal called *Chittra*. It is the fibre of Reissner. Its function is not yet known. It is also know as '*Brahma-nadi*.'"

While Rele plausibly identifies Reissner's fiber with the *Vajra nadi*, he mistakenly calls the fiber a nerve, mistakenly places the *Vajra nadi* within the *Chittra nadi*, and mistakenly asserts that the *Vajra nadi* is equivalent to the *Brahma nadi*. Nevertheless, Rele's identification of Reissner's fiber with the *Vajra nadi* would seemingly have established it as the central axis of *kundalini* yoga. However, instead, Rele concluded that "Kundalini, or serpent power as it is called is the Vagus nerve of modern times." This identification of *kundalini* with the vagus nerve, a paired nerve that wanders from the medulla to the carotid arteries and vocal cords, to the heart and lungs, and to the liver, spleen, stomach, and intestines, bears little resemblance to the textual descriptions of *kundalini*'s ascent through the concentric *Sushumna*, *Vajra*, *Chittra*, and *Brahma nadis* in the center of the spine.

Woodroffe wrote the foreword to Rele's book. He praised his scientific inquiry into yoga because, like Rele, he believed that there are lost secrets contained in ancient texts. However, Woodroffe disputed Rele's identification of *kundalini* with the vagus nerve, because, in his view, the *kundalini* is not composed of the gross substance of neural tissue, but "its Ground Substance." Also, he urged a closer adherence to the actual anatomical descriptions found in ancient texts. Like Vivekananda, Rele had uncovered ancient descriptions of the yoga anatomy that clearly correspond to the anatomy of Reissner's fiber.

After having located the source of the sleeping *kundalini* at the level of the conus medullaris, the distal swelling of the spinal cord that surrounds the terminal ventricle, Rele goes on to write:

> From this sleeping Kundalini, otherwise called Kula Kundali, there is described as extending a fibre which descends and shines in the cavity of Mula-lotus (Mooladara chakra) like a chain of brilliant lights. From the skirts of this dormant Kula-Kundali there starts another Kundalini, which ascends, along the Sushumna nadi and reaches ... to a point (Bindu or ParaSiva), which is bathed in the stream of ambrosia (Cerebrospinal-fluid) from the Eternal Bliss (Brahma-randhra), and illuminates even the lowermost cavity with her radiance.

Stripped of its obscuring metaphors such as "a chain of brilliant lights," "the stream of ambrosia," and "Eternal Bliss," the above passage describes the *kundalini* as ascending from the cavity of the *Mooladara chakra* through the *Sushumna nadi* to the *Brahma-randhra*, which is filled with CSF. The triangular-shaped *Mooladara chakra* at the end of the central canal in the conus medullaris is the terminal ventricle. The *Sushumna nadi* is the central canal. The *Brahma-randhra*, as defined by Rele, "is the cavity lying between the four inter-communicating ventricles of the brain and is continuous with the central canal of the *Sushumna nadi*, i.e., the spinal cord, known in Yogic literature as *Chittra*." The pathway of *kundalini* from the terminal ventricle through the central canal to the cerebral ventricle is the pathway of Reissner's fiber. Rele's interpretation of the yogic texts points toward Reissner's fiber, but as we follow Rele along the path that led him to identify the *kundalini* with the vagus nerve, we can almost feel the Devil's invisible presence shaping Rele's thoughts and opinions while professing that his supreme goal is bring about the "destruction of Superstition." The lost secrets of ancient interoceptions of Reissner's fiber that had been buried beneath layers of distortions and disguisings were, after thousands of years, about to make their connection with sixty-year-old objective scientific observations of the fiber. But the Devil had other plans.

Rele arrived at his puzzling identification of *kundalini* with the vagus nerve from his premise that *kundalini* yoga is "a science of physical and mental exercises of a particular form by which an individual establishes a conscious control over his autonomic nervous system so as to get in tune with the Infinite." This definition of *kundalini* yoga was inspired by a demonstration by Yogi Deshbandhu that he had witnessed as a medical student in Bombay. Deshbandhu stopped his heartbeat, split a hair with an arrow shot from twenty feet away, and broke an iron chain three-eighths of an inch in thickness with a single tug. Rele was especially curious about the physiology underlying the yogi's control over his cardiovascular system. He and a physician from the Bombay Medical Union examined the yogi's feats using stethoscopes, X-rays, and electrocardiography. These tests showed that during voluntary stoppages of the heart, it contracted and its apex moved internally about two-thirds of an inch from its normal position. While his pulse was impalpable and his heartbeat was inaudible, the rhythmic activity of his heart was recorded by the EKG. The yogi was also able to stop either his right or left radial pulse.

Searching for an answer, Rele concluded that voluntary control of the autonomic nervous system's regulation of cardiac activity achieved through the practice of yoga was the explanation of the yogi's remarkable feats. Exploring the philosophy underlying yoga, Rele learned that conquering desire, *Vasana*, liberates the soul from the vicious cycles of karma and rebirth. Conscious control of psychophysiological functions that are ordinarily controlled by the subconscious can "open the door to Liberation." Consciousness can expand into the eternal realm of the subconscious, "the presiding deity of the body." "On the physical plane," Rele writes, "this can only be done by controlling the cord of desire, the Vagus nerve (Kundalini), *i.e.* by consciously controlling all the involuntary actions of the body, which are more or less under the control of the Vagus nerve."

Loosely interpreting various textual descriptions, which locate the dormant *kundalini* somewhere between the navel and the penis, Rele concludes that the dormant *kundalini* is located in the solar plexus and connects below with the pelvic plexus near the rectum. It ascends through the cardiac, pharyngeal, and the cavernous plexus at the base of the skull and its nasociliary extensions that innervate the iris and the space between the eyebrows. Ultimately, it arrives at the *Brahma-randhra*, "a cavity in the brain where the Brahma, *i.e.* the Soul, is located, and the knowledge of which the yogi seeks to attain." Rele explains that the *Brahma-randhra* is the ventricular cavity above and continuous with the central canal. Here again, Rele illuminates Reissner's fiber's pathway, but turns away to make a fuzzy connection between the *Brahma-randhra* and the vagus nerve by noting that it originates, in part, from the floor of the fourth ventricle. To reconcile the fact that there are two vagus nerves, a right and left, with the textual descriptions of a single pathway of *kundalini* through the *Sushumna nadi*, Rele proposed that yogis recognized that the right vagus nerve has more efferent fibers than the left and therefore disregarded the left vagus nerve. To reconcile the fact that the *kundalini* travels through the *Sushumna nadi*, which Rele identifies with the spinal cord, with the fact that the vagus nerve wanders away from the spinal cord, Rele notes that the "plexuses throw out filaments to the Sushumna nadi."

The anatomy of the vagus nerve is not only inconsistent with descriptions of the yogic anatomy, but its physiology is ill suited to play its role as the *kundalini*. In the final chapter of *Mysterious Kundalini*, Rele discusses the paranormal and supernatural levels purportedly attained by yogis. According to Rele's interpretation of yogic texts, yoga masters can liberate their souls from their physical bodies to function in an "Astral body" formed by "Akasa material," the supersensible substrate of material reality. From this "Astral body" the yogi can withdraw his soul to the physical body "along a fine filament of ethereal substance which connects these two bodies together."

Rele offers little explanation of how the vagus nerve creates this connection. He writes, "In these perfections, or Siddhis, Kundalini does not take any part directly, but it does prepare the ground for the soul to vibrate through another channel than the nerves." He offers no suggestion as to what that other channel might be. His identification of the *Akasa* with the subarachnoid space, the space containing spidery filaments of connective tissue and CSF located between the delicate pia mater covering the brain and spinal cord and the fibrous arachnoid mater above it, is implausible and therefore widens the gap between *Siddhis*, *kundalini*, and *Akasa*. While yoga's claims of paranormal abilities strain our credulity, the direct consciousness and volitional control of macroscopic quantum events in Reissner's fiber provides a possible bridge between yoga and neuroscience.

Analyzing the various methods of yoga—postures (*asanas* and *mudras*), forceful muscular contractions (*bandhas*), and rhythmic breathing (*pranyama*)—Rele concludes that they are all methods of controlling the vagus nerve. Contractions of various muscles and bodily stretches are said to stimulate or inhibit vagal activity. Pressure on the center of the perineum exerted by the heel, for example, is said to block the downward efferent impulses of the pelvic plexus while leaving the upward impulses unchecked. Breath-holding stimulates vagal activity by increasing the venosity of the blood. An extreme example of these methods is exemplified by *Khechari Mudra*, the "King amongst the Mudras." Here, the yogi rolls his tongue upward and backward to close the larynx after a deep inhalation and thereby prevent exhalation. Inhibition of the vagus nerve caused by stimulation of nerves in the buccal cavity results in a forceful contraction of the heart. Thus, bottling up the energy absorbed by the tissues from the oxygenated blood, the yogi "can liberate this energy for action at his own sweet will. To all outward appearances a Yogi practicing this Mudra appears to be dead, and in this condition he can remain as long as he likes either buried under the earth or above it."

While interpretations of the methods of yoga are dubiously connected with the physiology of the vagus nerve, those methods are consistent with creating a patent central canal. Typically, the central canal becomes occluded during adulthood. This would correspond to the various knots or *grandhis* of the *sushumna nadi* described by *kundalini* yoga. *Asanas*, which twist and stretch the spine, could help remove occlusions in the central canal. Breathing exercises known as *pranyamas* combined with forceful muscular contractions or *bandhas* can produce pressurized waves of CSF directed toward the opening of the central canal. These are the "water hammer" waves proposed by the renowned neurosurgeon Dr. James Gardner to explain the dilations in the central canal that occur in syringomyelia. Anesthesiologists, following neurosurgical repair of the membranes surrounding the brain, produce similar pressurized waves to ensure that there are no leaks. By forcing expiration against a closed glottis (Valsalva maneuver), the anesthesiologist replicates a variation of the yoga practice of *pranyama* and *bandha*.

The devil ultimately thwarted Rele's journey to the convergence of ancient interoceptions of Reissner's fiber and modern objective observations. Rather than kindle the "Fire of Knowledge" with the mental friction of new ideas, Rele's convoluted tangle of poetic metaphors, misguided anatomical correspondences, and dubious neurophysiology further obscured the parallels between yoga and neuroscience in dark clouds. Apparently not content with twisting Rele's efforts into a tangled web that concealed the convergence of Reissner's fiber and innermost *nadis* of *kundalini* yoga, the devil pushed Rele's thoughts from reality. In 1931, Rele published *Vedic Gods as Figures of Biology*. Here, Rele proposes that the Vedic gods are actually representations of neuroanatomical structures. According Rele, because of prohibitions against dissections, ancient Vedic seers secretly carried corpses to lakes or rivers and submerged them. Over periods of days and weeks, they peeled off layers of decomposing flesh to reveal the nervous system which was similarly investigated by this method of fractional dissection. The Vedic gods are, according to Rele, metaphors of decomposing brains.

From this peculiar perspective, the fibers of the vagus nerve become the chariots on which Usas, the goddess of the dawn, rides. "The mention of the dawn as the first harbinger of life and as extending over five regions reaching far and wide," writes Rele, "shows the extent of the nerve (vagus) on which Usas ride." Reissner's fiber as the innermost *nadi* interocepted by ancient yogis sinks beneath the murky depths of waters filled with decomposing corpses reflecting poetic metaphorical images of Vedic gods.

Theos Bernard: "White Lama," Tantric Yogi

Shortly after Rele had identified *kundalini* with the right vagus nerve, Theos Bernard, the first doctoral student in religious studies at Columbia University, son of Glen Bernard, who had abandoned Theo as an infant to pursue "Yogic Science," and nephew of the flamboyant Pierre Bernard, aka Oom the Omnipotent, founder of the New York Sanskrit College in midtown Manhattan and The Mystic Order of the Tantriks of India at the Clarkstown Country Club in Nyack, New York, was establishing himself as a celebrity by feeding America's hunger for exotic spiritual truths from the East. Rejecting the West's "preconceived notion that man cannot know metaphysical truths by direct experience," and "therefore, at best, metaphysical truths can only be speculations, inferences, or ungrounded faith," Bernard sought to know those truths directly. He traveled to India and Tibet in search of an authentic Tantric yogi who could teach him to become one. His goal was to realize yoga's mission to unite the human with the divine.

Using his charm and sincere dedication to learn Tantric yoga, Bernard eventually became the first Westerner to gain entrance to the forbidden city of Lhasa in Tibet, which had sealed its borders to foreigners 250 years earlier. There, he was initiated into the inner circle of Tantra yoga by the highest lama in Tibet.

After years of arduous practice, Bernard exulted over the "deep joys that I had never before dreamt existed in this life." Wishing to ground his personal experience in the nascent field of biological psychiatry, Bernard searched for the neuroanatomical basis of Tantric yoga.

In 1936, Bernard met Rele in India. A self-described skeptic, Bernard wrote in his journal that "every expert had the ultimate answer" and "filled their baskets with plucked finalities from the teetering tree of prejudice." His credo was "study everything, accept nothing." He realized that Rele's description of the *kundalini*'s ascent along the plexuses of the sympathetic nervous system and its identification with the right vagus nerve bears almost no resemblance to traditional yogic texts. If those texts are based on interoceptions of neurophysiological events during altered states of consciousness, then Reissner's fiber is the true pathway of *kundalini*. In *Heaven Lies Within Us*, published in 1939, which told of his adventures and explorations of yoga, Bernard wrote, "Inside this central (*Sushumna*) nadi, the Yogi identifies an invisible nadi known in the West as the fibre of Reissner, but which is known here as *Chittra* (the Heavenly Passage, in Sanskrit)." Bernard lifted Rele's obscure footnote about Reissner's fiber to its justified place as the tangible intersection between lost secrets of yoga and modern neuroscience.

Bernard's adventures captured the public's imagination. In 1937, his exploits appeared on the front page of the *New York Times*. He proclaimed that he was the reincarnation of Padmasambhava, the saint and Tantric master who had brought Tantric Buddhism to Tibet during the eighth century. He would be the spiritual savior of humankind. Lost between his grandiose claims and the authentic teachings of Tantric yoga was the scientific hypothesis that the *Chittra nadi*, the "Heavenly Passage" interocepted by yogis in altered states of consciousness, and Reissner's fiber observed under the microscope were the same.

In 1947 while searching for a rare manuscript in the hills of Spiti, India, Bernard was rumored to have been attacked by Lahouli tribesmen. He was never seen again.

According to one of his biographers, Paul Hackett, Bernard was on a quest to find a manuscript documenting Jesus's "lost years" between the ages of 14 and 30 when he learned about yoga. The basis for Bernard's belief was accounts by three individuals who claimed to have read the manuscript. In 1894, Nicholas Notovitch published *The Unknown Life of Jesus Christ* that detailed his travels to the Hemis Monastery in Leh, Ladakh. There he claims to have read a Tibetan translation of a document about Jesus's studies of Hinduism and Buddhism, proving that Christianity is not a "Jewish thing." In 1909, Levi H. Dowling, a preacher who had served in the American Civil War, published *The Aquarian Gospel of Jesus* which made similar claims while announcing the coming of the "Age of Aquarius." In 1929, Swami Abhedananda published his accounts of his retracing of Notovitch's journey to Hemis Monastery. He also claimed to have read the manuscript and made his own translation.

While in India, Bernard met with the Russian artist and mystic Nicholas Roerich who suggested that Bernard could find the manuscript by visiting the Ki Monastery in western Tibet. Had either Roerich or Bernard read the account of the missionary A.H. Francke's visit to the Ki Monastery, Bernard might have been saved from his fateful encounter with the Lahouli. Francke had documented that the monastery had been ransacked during the Dogra war. All the books and manuscripts had been destroyed.

Forced to take an alternate route on their return from the Ki Monastery by torrential rains and massive snowfalls, Bernard and his companion crossed a chain suspension bridge on ponies. Bernard and his party of Muslim porters were attacked by Lahouli tribesmen who follow a combination of Hinduism and Tibetan Buddhism. A gunman fired a fatal shot at Bernard. Fearing that his companion would be a witness to the murder, the gunman killed him too. Theos Bernard's legacy quickly faded.

It was somewhat revived in the twenty-first century after Hackett, as a college student, stumbled upon Bernard's *Penthouse of the Gods – A Pilgrimage Into the Heart of Tibet and the Sacred City of Lhasa* in a used bookstore. Initially believing the book to be "yet another pseudo-Orientalist travelogue," he eventually saw Bernard as an important figure in American religious history who had been cast into the dustbin of history. While Hackett retrieved fascinating and lurid details of Bernard's self-promotion and seductions, and his adventures and spiritual journey, his identification of Reissner's fiber as the tangible intersection between lost secrets of yoga and modern neuroscience, between the human and the divine, remains forgotten.

The fading echoes of Bernard's proposed identification of Reissner's fiber with the *Chittra nadi* were drowned out by a growing chorus of yogis and swamis led by the ghost of Vivekananda. In 1959, Swami Vishnu-devananda wrote *The Complete Illustrated Book of Yoga*, which greatly enhanced yoga's credibility in the West. In his explanation of how yogis open the *Sushumna nadi* through breathing exercises, he uses the exact words used by Vivekananda in his London speech about the canal "closed at the lower end, which is situated near what is called the sacral plexus." He then goes on to follow Vivekananda's proposal that the *chakras* correspond to the nerve plexuses above the sacral plexus by tentatively proposing that the prostatic, solar, cardiac, laryngeal, and cavernous plexuses correspond to the *chakras* that ascend from the *Mooladara chakra* and are aligned with the *Sushumna nadi*. Paramahansa Yogananda, whose book *Autobiography of a Yogi* has sold more than four million copies and inspired worldwide interest in Hindu spirituality, similarly identified the *chakras* with various plexuses. In his book *God Talks With Arjuna: The Bhagavad Gita*, Yogananda states:

> The yogi reverses the searchlights of intelligence, mind and life force inward through a secret astral passage, the coiled way of the kundalini in the coccygeal plexus, and upward through the sacral, the lumbar, and the higher dorsal, cervical, and medullary plexuses, and the spiritual eye at the point between the eyebrows, to reveal finally the soul's presence in the highest center (sahasrara) in the brain.

Attesting to the depths of oblivion to which Bernard's identification of the *Chittra nadi* with Reissner's fiber has sunk are the recent investigations of two researchers of *kundalini* yoga, Gopi Krishna and Hiroshi Motoyama.

Gopi Krishna, who, after prolonged meditation, experienced what he believes to have been an awakening of *kundalini*:

> Suddenly, with a roar like that of a waterfall, I felt a stream of liquid light entering my brain through the spinal cord. ... I was no longer myself, or to be more accurate, no longer as I knew myself to be, a small point of awareness confined to a body, but instead was a vast circle of consciousness in which the body was but a point, bathed in light and in a state of exultation and happiness impossible to describe.

Krishna recognized that the diagrams and descriptions of the yoga anatomy initially strike the scientific mind as "entirely unscientific and irrational, the fanciful creation of deluded authorities or of unscrupulous charlatans to deceived the credulous." Currently, the truth about *kundalini* "lies concealed under the cloak of weird formulations, fantastic creations and mythical beings." Given our ancient ancestors' ignorance of physiology and the "superstitious awe with which the inexplicable phenomena relating to the mind and body were regarded," it is not surprising that the possible neuroanatomical basis of *kundalini* yoga remains obscure. Current accounts seduce credulous seekers of the supernatural.

Seeking to establish the groundwork for a scientific understanding of *kundalini* yoga, Krishna writes that the "whole vast structure of Kundalini yoga revolves around" the *Brahma-randhra*, the Cave of Brahma, which he, like Rele, identifies as the cerebrospinal fluid-filled cavity above and continuous with the central canal. Like Rele, he also illuminates the pathway along which Reissner's fiber descends from below the pineal gland, through the third and fourth ventricles of the brain, and down the central canal. But the fiber is unseen.

While Krishna's identification of the *Sushumna nadi* with the central canal is consistent with yogic texts, his physiological explanation of the awakening of the *kundalini* and its ascent through the central canal is as implausible as Vivekanada's:

> It was obvious that by some mysterious process the precious secretion of the seminal glands was drawn up into the spinal tube and through the interlinking nerves transferred into a subtle essence, then distributed to the brain and the vital organs, darting across the nerve filaments and the spinal cord to reach them.

Dr. Hiroshi Motoyama, who reported experiences of *kundalini* awakening and measured electrical and biophotonic from the *chakras*, argued that while the identification of the *Sushumna nadi* with the central canal "sounds plausible at first," it is "difficult to accept" because "the central canal of the spinal cord contains no nerve fibers, only cerebro-spinal fluid." However, while it is true that the central canal contains neither axons nor dendrites, it is not true that it contains only cerebrospinal fluid. It contains Reissner's fiber. Departing from Rele's and Krishna's interpretation of the yogic texts, Motoyama refers to the *Brahma-randhra* as an opening at the top of the skull and concludes, "It is also neurologically impossible for the spinal cord to have an opening at the top of the head for in the inflow and outflow of prana," aka *kundalini*. Rejecting the correspondence between the *Sushumna nadi* and the central canal, Motoyama proposes that it corresponds to the Governing Vessel, the central meridian of the acupuncture anatomy.

Motoyama developed an instrument (Apparatus for Meridian Identification) to establish the meridians of acupuncture by measuring the electrical conductivity between acupuncture points. While Motoyama's studies are suggestive of the possibility that acupuncture points and meridians are electrically distinguishable, these studies do not provide an anatomical basis for them. Motoyama's identification of the *Sushumna nadi* with the Governing Vessel rather than the central canal, therefore, does not contribute to an anatomical understanding of yoga or acupuncture and derives from the error that the central canal contains nothing but cerebrospinal fluid.

Rele's identification of the *Vajra nadi* with Reissner's fiber and Bernard's identification with the *Chittra nadi* remain under the Devil's cloak. Reissner's fiber as a tightrope across the abyss separating *kundalini* yoga and neuroscience remains a road not traveled.

Reissner's Fiber and Acupuncture as Applied Taoism

Written descriptions of the subtle anatomy appeared in *The Yellow Emperor's Classic of Internal Medicine*, composed between 475 BCE and 220 CE. While the Chinese subtle anatomy was rooted in Taoism and was described as a means towards achieving spiritual enlightenment, most texts dealt with its applications to medicine. Various ailments were treated by directing the flow of *Qi* along various meridians by stimulating acupuncture points on the skin.

Interest in acupuncture declined during the seventeenth century. Regarding acupuncture as an irrational superstition, the Emperor excluded it from the Imperial Medical Institute in 1822. As Chinese medicine became increasingly westernized, it eventually was outlawed along with other traditional forms of Chinese medicine in 1929. It was revived in 1949 by the Communist government.

The path from traditional teachings about acupuncture to Reissner's fiber started around 1957 in North Korea. The leader and founding father of North Korea, Kim Il Sung, grandfather of the current leader of North Korea, Kim Jung Un, instituted a new policy to establish research institutes to study the scientific basis of traditional Chinese medicine which was renamed "Oriental medicine." One of the leaders of this movement was Bong Han Kim. In 1940, he graduated from the Medical School of Kyungsung University, in what is now South Korea, and later worked in the physiology department there. During the Korean War, under circumstances that are unclear, Kim moved to North Korea. There, in 1957, he became Chief for Physiological Lectures at the Pyungyang Medical School.

In 1961, at the Pyungyang Medical School Scientific symposium, Kim presented his findings, titled *Research on the Real Entity of Kyungrak (Meridian) System*, which announced the discovery of the anatomical basis of acupuncture meridians. He demonstrated a previously unknown system of ducts, corpuscles, and fluid that would come to be known as Bonghan ducts, corpuscles, and liquor, which comprise the Bonghan system. When asked how he discovered this system while so many others had failed, he replied that his absolute belief in its existence inspired him to persevere in spite of thousands of failures.

In 1962, Kim Il Sung sent Kim a congratulatory note, stating, "Bong Han Kim has significantly contributed to establishing solid scientific and tangible evidence for the theory of Oriental medicine, Korea has kept for centuries, and to the progresses in modern biology and medical sciences." The following year, supplied by the North Korean government with cutting edge optical and electron microscopes, and radioisotope and other tracers, Kim developed his research. He showed a vast distribution of Bonghan ducts and showed that the Bonghan corpuscles contained "sanals" that possessed properties of stem cells. His work was hailed as a "monumental theory in global science," comparable to the Nobel Prize winning discoveries of Ivan Pavlov. His work was translated into several languages and distributed throughout the world. The Democratic People's Republic of Korea's Communist Party greatly expanded the scale of Kim's research, establishing the Kyungrak Research Institute with over 40 laboratories. Kim was its president and he was awarded the People's Award, the highest scientific honor in North Korea.

Then, in 1966, the Kyungrak Research Institute was suddenly shut down. Kim's publications were banned and he mysteriously disappeared. Various theories have been proposed regarding the sudden fall of Bong Han Kim, including questions about the legitimacy of his methods and results. Because Kim's publications were reports rather than peer-reviewed scientific articles that require detailed description of methods, his investigations have been difficult to replicate.

According to Hyun Sik Kim, who defected from North Korea, and who worked as a tutor for Kim Il Sung's children and was friends with an associate of Bong Han Kim, Bong Han was a victim of a political struggle. Keum Chul Park, who was second in command of the Communist Party in the Democratic People's Republic of Korea, was using Kim's fame for political gain. He provided Kim with almost unlimited financial support and the best scientists in North Korea. He also began planning an International Kyungrak Symposium with the intention of promoting Kim's work for a future Nobel Prize. Translators for Russian, Chinese, Japanese, English, French, and German languages were recruited. Hyun Sik Kim, a professor in Russian language, was selected as the Russian translator.

Feeling politically threatened, Kim Il Sung began a campaign of discrediting Kim and Park. He enlisted a group of scientists who were jealous of Kim's fame to criticize his research as fraudulent. He accused Park of promoting Kim's deceptions for political gain, using an aggressive media campaign to convince his followers that Kim was a South Korean spy sent to discredit North Korean science. Following Kim's banishment, Park was removed from power.

The key experiment that pointed toward Reissner's fiber as the central axis of the subtle anatomy that underlies acupuncture is the following: Kim injected radioactive phosphorous (P^{32}) into acupuncture points on a rabbit's abdomen corresponding to the Governing Vessel and traced its flow using autoradiography. The isotopes labeled a threadlike duct inside the central canal. Kim named it the "neural Bonghan duct." Injections into other sites dispersed. Consistent with Kim's experiments are the observations of G. Erbl-Roth. In 1951, this German researcher succeeded in collecting fresh specimens of the fiber from mammals and found that the fiber was hollow. Kim made no reference to Reissner's fiber, but by identifying the Governing Vessel with a fiber within the central canal, Kim shifted Motoyoma's identification of the *Sushumna nadi* with the Governing Vessel from an abstract level to a physical level.

For 45 years following Kim's disappearance, his work was obscured by a cloud of conspiracy theories. Then, in 2000, Kwang Sop Soh, a physicist at Seoul National University, established the Biomedical Physics Laboratory for Korean Medicine to explore the physiological basis of Oriental medicine. He measured specific electronic, photonic, and acoustic properties of meridians and acupuncture points, but soon realized that his findings demanded an anatomical substrate. Recalling Kim's reports on the Bonghan system that he had read as a graduate student in physics at the University of Kansas in 1970, Soh attempted to replicate his findings. In collaboration with Satoru Fujiwara, a Japanese scientist who had replicated Kim's work during the 1960s, Soh "rediscovered" the Bonghan system. He has gone on to develop new imaging techniques based on fluorescent magnetic nanoparticles and confocal laser scanning microscopy, and has been a catalyst for establishing research centers around the world to investigate the revolutionary implications of the Bonghan system. In 2004, Soh proposed that Bonghan ducts act as optical channels for coherent biophotons. In 2009, at the urging of the South Korean government, Soh and colleagues renamed the Bonghan system because of its associations with North Korean politics. Its new name is the Primo vascular system.

In 2008, Byung-Cheon Lee, a member of Soh's laboratory, reported the existence of a novel threadlike structure in the cerebral ventricle and central canal of rabbits. While Lee does not refer to Kim's discovery of the "neural Bonghan duct," he does address the critical question of whether the novel threadlike structure he observed is Reissner's fiber. He rejects this identification because the threadlike structure he observed has "nodes," "corpuscles," and "branches," and its diameter is 30 micrometers compared to the reported 4 micrometer diameter of Reissner's fiber. However, Reissner's fiber's rapid postmortem degeneration and markedly variable responses to preservation and imaging techniques has made precise characterization extremely difficult. For 40 years after its discovery, the scientific consensus was that Reissner's fiber was an artifact. Its existence was disputed by leading anatomists for another 20 years. Lee's method of dissecting the fourth ventricle of a brain mildly cooled on an aluminum foil-covered ice pack, introducing hematoxylin drop by drop for several minutes, introducing buffered saline in a similar manner, removing the choroids plexus, sectioning the threadlike structure and staining it with DNA specific dyes followed by phospholipids specific dyes created fertile ground for introducing artifactual errors. Furthermore, "nodes," "corpuscles," and "branches" have been observed in Reissner's fiber. The most important evidence pointing toward the identity of Reissner's fiber and the novel threadlike structure observed by Lee is the absence of Reissner's fiber from Lee's observations and the absence of observations of an additional novel threadlike structure in the central canal from any of the reports from investigators of Reissner's fiber from 1860 to the present. Almost 150 years after its discovery, Reissner's fiber continues to play the Devil's trick of convincing people that it doesn't exist.

Kim named the corpuscles of the Bonghan system "sanals" or "living eggs" which he claimed have regenerative properties. Soh and his associates renamed "sanals" as "Primo microcells" and created a new term "primogenesis" to describe the regenerative properties of these structures. "Sanals" and "Primo microcells" correspond to exosomes, which have been implicated in neurogenesis, and to the membrane-bounded spherical bodies within Reissner's fiber.

By providing evidence for the empirical basis of the Governing Vessel, Kim and his followers have shown how traditional Chinese medicine and acupuncture as applied Taoism can converge with modern science. However, currently the spurious distinctions between the neural Bonghan duct, the novel threadlike structure inside the central canal, and Reissner's fiber have created diverging paths. The attempt to identify the Governing Vessel with a physical structure that is unseen when Reissner's fiber is seen and seen only when the fiber is unseen perpetuates the status of the central meridian of acupuncture as a primitive, metaphysical abstraction.

Personal Encounters with Reissner's Fiber as the Devil According to Baudelaire

In 1970, during my junior year of college, after having found intellectual certainty in mathematics and physics, I encountered the Heisenberg's Uncertainty Principle and Gödel's Incompleteness Theorem. Having learned that my scientific road to Truth had reached an impasse, I, fueled by the wave of Eastern mysticism and psychedelicism, wondered if yoga's claims of knowing the means of reaching the Absolute Truth were true. Specifically, I wanted to see if there was a quantum biophysical circuit in the central nervous system corresponding to the yoga anatomy. Wishing to ground my quixotic quest in a career path, I decided to go to medical school. There, I met the Chairman of the Neuroscience Department, University of Connecticut Health Center, Dr. Charles Loeser.

I met him at a student faculty party the night before my first day of classes. His slightly disheveled hair, "UCONN STAPH" sweatshirt, and humble, amiable manner invited me tell him my dreams. I told him of my frustration with physics' abandonment of reality for clouds of probability. How biology worked with the outdated Bohr atom. Then as my dreams entered the twilight zone where New Age quantum woo, the psychedelic world, and science intersect, I timorously told him of my interest in the parallels between the philosophical implications of modern physics and Eastern mysticism. As my words, "I, uh ... have been wondering if the anatomy described by yogis might correspond to quantum biophysical systems in the central nervous system," hung in the air, Dr. Loeser smiled and invited me to his lab.

A revolving darkroom door delivered me into another world. Darkening shades and patches of aluminum foil covered the windows, shutting out the light so that stray photons would not interfere with the instruments. Digital LED readouts from silent black instruments flickered with a reddish glow. A large metal cylinder surrounded by various exotic attachments and tangles of multicolored wires dominated from the room's center. Dr. Loeser explained that the device was a time-resolved ultra-fast fluorescent microscope that analyzed quantum biological events by measuring the decay time of excited molecules.

Funding for the equipment was provided by a grant from the Army. They wanted to better understand the pathophysiology of malaria. After having quickly satisfied the Army's requirements, Dr. Loeser focused on more interesting projects. An earlier project had investigated quantum mechanical effects involving LSD and serotonergic receptors. When he told me, with a wry smile, that he had to fill out a lot of federal paperwork to explain a "dilution error," I knew he was fellow psychedelic traveler. Currently he was investigating the interface between cancer cells and antibodies. This project had personal significance for him. He had undergone radical neck surgery to treat a malignant melanoma.

Returning to Dr. Loeser's brightly lit office, with my quantum mystical dreams searching for a tangible connection, I quickly got to the point: is there a hollow tube that runs through the center of the brain and spinal cord that corresponds to the *Sushumna nadi*? My question focused his accumulated knowledge on Reissner's fiber. But, playing its role as the Devil according to Baudelaire, it wasn't there.

Dr. Loeser smiled and told me about a hollow passageway that runs through the center of the spinal cord called the central canal. Textbooks described it as a typically occluded remnant of embryological development. But for Dr. Loeser and me, it was now illuminated by the twilight glow where science and mysticism intersect.

Dr. Loeser, for whom an eponymous award is now given annually to "the faculty member who has the ability to evoke in students an enthusiasm for learning, a desire to emulate their own attributes of scholarly curiosity, and to give wholeheartedly to advance the welfare and education of their students," then took me on a magical tour of the central canal. Pulling *Gray's Anatomy* from his shelf, he showed me how the poppy seed-sized ball of cells implanted on the uterine wall flattens and stretches. Then a faint streak running from head to toe deepens into a groove. The banks on either side of this neural groove began to thicken and rise. They arch toward each other. Eventually, the rising, arching crests fuse to form a hollow tube, the neural tube, the forerunner of the central canal. The symmetric tube polarizes. The anterior portion swells to become the brain and the posterior stretched to become the spinal cord. The ends of the neural tube close and CSF replaces the amniotic fluid that had previously flowed through it. Pressure from the CSF triggers tension and stretch receptors along the inner walls, which sent signals to the proliferating cells of the developing brain. Chemicals secreted into the CSF promoted further growth and development. The brain expands 100,000-fold as the fluid-filled cavity in the center of the developing central nervous system stretches, bulges, and contorts to create an interconnected network of fluid-filled chambers and passageways called the neurocele. The finished product is a system of fluid-filled spaces inside the brain called the cerebral ventricles and a narrow passageway running through the entire length of the spinal cord called the central canal.

Seven weeks after conception, when the embryo is the size of a grain of rice and looks like a tiny seahorse with a bulging head, gill-like slits, and a face like a beluga whale, secretions from the floor and roof of the fluid-filled central chamber in the center of the embryonic brain known as the diencephalon coalesce into a barely visible thread called Reissner's fiber. But this was not part of the tour. It was concealed by the Devil's loveliest trick.

With the central canal now glowing with the lost secrets of the *Sushumna nadi*, Dr. Loeser next took me on a historical tour of another lost secret, the CSF. While the presence of five ounces of clear fluid surrounding the adult brain and spinal cord and filling its hollow cavities and passageways would seem hard to miss, it was not until the eighteenth century that the existence CSF became an established fact. According to some historians, Imhotep, the physician and architect of ancient Egypt, was the first person to document observations of the CSF. In 1862, the Egyptologist Edwin Smith discovered a papyrus, dated 1600 BC, which contained a reprint of Imhotep's discovery made in 3000 BC. Here, the ancient Egyptian physician described a case of head trauma which resulted in a fluid flowing from the interior of the head.

While Hippocrates (460–375 BC), when describing congenital hydrocephalus, commented on "water" surrounding the brain, and Galen (130–200) referred to "excremental liquid" in the ventricles of the brain that is purged into the nose, subsequent anatomists missed it for sixteen centuries. The practice of cutting off the head of the deceased while in an upright position, and the Church's promotion of Galen's belief that the ventricles contained a vaporous spiritual substance, contributed to late scientific confirmation of the existence of CSF.

Medieval philosophers and Church fathers adopted Galen's view. Owing to the dominating influence of religion over science during those times, anatomists adopted it as well. They referred to "animal spirits"—derived from the Latin word for "mind," *anima*—"that flow through the ventricles."

During the Renaissance, Galen's view fell out of favor. The leading neuroanatomist of the seventeenth century and the father of clinical neuroanatomy, Thomas Willis, referred to the ventricles as "vile places, sewers for the carrying away of excreted matter," mistakenly believing them to contain "foul vapors."

It wasn't until the late 1730s that Swedenborg rediscovered CSF. But because Swedenborg expressed his findings in abstruse philosophical and theological language, and because he had no academic affiliations or scientific correspondents, his discovery went unrecognized, and his work was shunned for over one hundred and fifty years. Swedenborg had rediscovered the spinal fluid in the course of searching for the anatomical seat of the soul, seeking the "soul in the temple wherein she dwells." During the course of his dissections, he encountered a "highly gifted juice" dispensed from the roof of the fourth ventricle that flowed into the third ventricle, the "womb of the virgin Mary."

While Dr. Loeser's evocation of Swedenborg's scientific and spiritual quest to find the anatomical seat of the soul fueled my faith in the reality of the subtle anatomy, his cryptic mystical foreshadowing of Reissner's fiber was obscured by the Devil's shadow. Dr. Loeser continued with his tour of the developing neurocele unaware of Swedenborg's warning: "For even though we know all things, still they are merely effects, for the entire product of the infinite forces flow forth from the potencies and principles of this fibril; and thus we really understand nothing if we are ignorant of this fibril in respect to its quality."

"Eventually, the diencephalon develops into a slit-like cavity in the center of the brain called the third ventricle whose walls are named thalami which comes from the Latin word for 'marriage chamber,'" Dr.

Loeser continued. "The floor is called the hypothalamus. Its roof, the epithalamus, means 'ode to the bride and groom.'"

The thalamus is taught to medical students as a relay station that sends sensory signals to the cerebral cortex. Its clinical significance is recognized because strokes involving the thalamus lead to syndromes manifested by pain, lethargy, and mood swings.

Following its poetic origins, the hypothalamus means beneath marriage chamber. This is appropriate because neurons of the hypothalamus secrete two hormones associated with love and lust into the third ventricle, oxytocin and vassopressin.

The epithalamus's most notable structure is the pineal gland, a reddish, pea-sized, pinecone-shaped body protruding from the rear wall of our third ventricle. Just bellow the pineal gland is the subcommissural organ. But concealed beneath the Devil's cloak, it was not part of the tour.

Although the pineal has been a target of metaphysical speculation since at least the second century, it is only recently that the modern mistaken characterization of the pineal gland as a vestigial remnant, whose primary utility was a calcified landmark for the midline on skull X-rays, has been corrected.

For more than fifteen centuries, physicians debated the pineal's possible role in regulating the flow of the volatile, vaporous spiritual substance believed to flow through the neurocele. During the seventeenth century, Rene Descartes, often credited as the father of Western philosophy, proposed that the pineal is seat of the soul, the locus of the will's influences on the motor pathways of the brain.

Anatomists have long been aware that in some lizards, frogs, and lampreys the pineal extends to the top of the skull as a functioning third eye known as the parietal eye. The lizard-like reptile tuatara's parietal eyes has a lens and retina. In some species of frogs, snakes, lizards, and fish, including tuna and sharks, the parietal eye is a visible light-sensitive spot on top of the head. The nineteenth-century theosophist Madame Blavatsky identified the pineal gland as the dormant "mystical third eye" described by ancient Hindus and Taoists. She attributed the mineralization of the gland to a fossilization of it spiritual capacities. Another theosophist, C.W. Leadbeater, claimed that by extending an "etheric tube" from the pineal gland one could develop extrasensory perceptions of astronomical and atomic phenomena.

Empirically based scientific studies of the pineal began in 1917 when scientists discovered that pineal extracts from cows lightened frog's skin. It was not until 1958, however, that Aaron Lerner at Yale, after analyzing 250,000 frozen cow pineal glands, identified the substance and named it "melatonin." Nobel Laureate Julius Axelrod then elucidated its role in human physiology. Its rhythms of secretion and their responses to light are correlated to sleep–wake cycles, seasonal affective disorders, and sexual development.

Recalling his knowledge of the biochemistry of the pineal and the pharmacology of LSD, and correctly guessing that visions of the "third eye" were occupying my thoughts, Dr. Loeser explained molecular similarities between LSD and melatonin. Sensing that my inner visions were expanding beyond even the twilight zone where mysticism, psychedelics, and science intersect, he brought me back by explaining the migration of neural stem cells from the developing neurocele to become the external sensory organs. I asked if the inner surface of the brain, the lining of the neurocele, might have sensory functions too. Dr. Loeser, once again, let his thoughts roam unfamiliar territory and explained some recent speculations about chemical pathways through the CSF between the pituitary gland and hypothalamus. Neither the neurosecretory pathway of Reissner's fiber discovered by Enami twenty years earlier, nor the inner-directed sensory system surrounding the fiber fifty years earlier, were part of the tour.

As the images of the developing embryo played in my mind, I imagined an inner-directed sensory system. Where it was looking, I could not say. Then, recalling the mystics' description of the oneness of reality beyond the duality of mind and matter and separation between inner and outer reality I imagined a universal theory of relativity according to which the illusory separation between inner and outer reality results from the embryological separation between the inner and outer surfaces of the brain. Reining in my soaring thoughts back to the bedrock of neuroanatomy, I next asked Dr. Loeser if there is a structure that might correspond to the triangular-shaped abode of the coiled sleeping *kundalini,* the *Mooladara chakra.*

Unaware of such a structure, Dr. Loeser thumbed through the pages of *Gray's Anatomy* and to his surprise learned of the terminal ventricle, which, curiously, like the *Mooladara chakra,* was described as triangular-shaped. Reissner's fiber, coiled within the terminal ventricle, was not part of the tour.

Eager to learn more about this enigmatic structure and to see if there are any features that might suggest it is the site of the sleeping *kundalini,* we prepared histological sections of a preserved human spinal cord at the level of the terminal ventricle. To our astonishment, we observed circular clusters of cells surrounding the terminal ventricle that are characteristic of secretory cells. After Dr. Loeser whimsically dubbed our discovery "Wile's hormone," I enthusiastically set out to identify it. After laboriously obtaining a specimen from a dog that had been sacrificed during a neurosurgical study of cerebral blood flow, my enthusiasm waned when I realized that I would need thousands of specimens.

Visions of a psychedelic explosion created by a mixing of Wile's hormone and endogenous psychedelics that would burst open the doors of perception fueled my quantum mystical dreams. But something was missing. Psychedelics can dissolve socially constructed filters and conditioning and thereby open the doors of perception. But if the mystical experiences of yogis are akin to psychedelic experiences, their purported paranormal powers would be illusions induced by hallucinations. The expansion of consciousness by psychedelics does not extend knowledge beyond the limits of science defined by the Uncertainty Principle and the Incompleteness Theorem. Something was missing.

Breaking the Devil's Spell

It had been nearly eighteen months since I had met Dr. Loeser and learned about the central canal, the pineal gland, and the terminal ventricle. Googling had not yet been invented. So, I spent countless hours in the library tracking down and photocopying articles I had found from bibliographies and searches using the massive volumes of *Index Medicus* that list biological journal articles according to key words. But Reissner's fiber was hiding from my investigations in plain sight. The Devil was using the rigid filters of the neuron doctrine paradigm to make it invisible.

I also pored over translations of yogic texts and books by modern yogis such as the *Complete Illustrated Book of Yoga* by Swami Vishnu Devananda and *Autobiography of a Yogi* by Yogananda. Shining through the fog of metaphranding and paraphranding images of thousand-petaled lotuses, elephants, hares, and the sun and moon were descriptions of subtle nerve tubes within the *Sushumna nadi* that I had previously identified with the central canal. The *Vajra*, *Chittra*, and *Brahma nadi* were said to be as subtle as a spider's thread, as thin as the hundredth part of the fiber in lotus stalks, or like unto the ten-millionth part of the end of a hair. With Reissner's fiber playing its trick of convincing neuroscientists that it didn't exist, I imagined the subtle innermost *nadis* to be the electron orbitals and subatomic particles of the molecules inside the central canal that were known through supersensory perceptions.

During those eighteen months, I came to know Dr. Loeser as an avatar of the archetype of the Trickster. The Trickster is the cunning, playful, wise fool who rebels against authority to reveal timeless truths hidden by socially constructed paradigms. Known in Greek mythology as Hermes, the messenger of the gods, the Trickster orchestrates synchronicities that meaningfully link our inner and outer worlds.

The guardians of the prevailing paradigm that had filtered Reissner's fiber from my intensive search rigidly and rigorously demanded strict adherence to its principles. As Tolstoy once observed:

> I know that most men, including those at ease with problems of the greatest complexity, can seldom accept even the simplest and most obvious truth if it be such as would oblige them to admit the falsity of conclusions which they have delighted in explaining to colleagues, which they have proudly taught to others, and which they have woven, thread by thread, into the fabric of their lives.

Dr. Loeser was different. As the Trickster, he encouraged a playful breaking of the boundaries of our ordinary perceptions of reality. He delighted in taking off the mask of petty authoritarians and making them play the fool. One time, an especially officious, pompous, ornery professor across the hall from Dr. Loeser returned to his office to find that his desk had been turned upside down. Under the circumstances, I thought it best to look down and hide my grin. But out of the corner of my eye, I could see an almost imperceptible mischievous grin briefly play across Dr. Loeser's lips.

Several days later, Dr. Loeser broke the Devil's spell. "You won't believe this," he beamed as he reached for a journal on his desk. "You dreamed it and here it is!" As I scanned the article titled "Studies concerning the function of the complex subcommissural organ-liquor fibre: The binding ability of the liquor fibre to pyrocatechin derivatives and its functional aspects," by a German scientist named Johann Hess, I felt as if my quixotic quantum mystical dreams had crystallized in the physical plane.

Had I glanced at the title of the article on the cover of the new issue of the journal *Brain Research*, which I routinely did as the new medical journals were placed on a table in the library, I would not have realized its significance. I was not aware that the term "liquor" derived from the little used synonym for the CSF, "liquor cerebrospinalis." But the term "liquor fibre" immediately aroused Dr. Loeser's playful curiosity.

Olry and Haines referred to Reissner's fiber as the Devil according to Baudelaire because it seemed to be a counterexample to the "never-ending updating of terms that had been coined by various researchers." But here, in a counterexample to Olry and Haines' assertion that Reissner's fiber has only been known as Reissner's fiber, the fiber escaped from the Devil's cloak as the crystallization of the obscure object of our quest. Rele's and Bernard's previous identifications of the fiber with the innermost *nadis* had faded so far into oblivion that it was not until 35 years later, after countless Google searches, I learned of them by first perusing the glossary in Rele's *Mysterious Kundalini* and then Bernard's *Heaven Lies Within Us.*

Reissner's fiber called to me like the Burning Bush proclaiming, "I am that I am." Fearing that the inspirational glow from that numinous revelation would be snuffed out by the avalanche of facts about the anatomy, histology, physiology, pathology, and pharmacology of the kidney and lungs that were poised to come crashing down on me for the rest of the semester, I pleaded with Dr. Loeser to arrange for me to postpone the remainder of classes and to pursue an independent research project to explore the fiber. Animated by the archetypal powers of the Trickster, Dr. Loeser was soon on the phone to an administrator at the National Marine Fisheries Service's Woods Hole Laboratories, gleefully informing him, "We'll be needing bench space and large tanks for some small sharks we'll be using." Responding to a slight hesitancy, Dr. Loeser channeled more energy into his Trickster persona. "We're no fly by night operation," he chortled. "We're funded by the United States Army!"

While arranging to move to Woods Hole, I contacted my college advisor, Willard Roth, who, I learned, had investigated the subcommissural organ as a professor at Harvard Medical School. In 1954, Professor Roth injected dyes and showed that the subcommissural is outside the blood brain barrier. During our telephone conversation, he told me, "These structures are pregnant with meaning, but I'm not meant to be their midwife."

Later, after learning about Rakic's studies of the subcommissural organ, I met with him to discuss Reissner's fiber. Lining the walls of his office were wooden boxes of microscope slides. Each contained dozens of microscopic slices of brains, from hundreds of monkeys and mice whose fetal brains had been labeled with radioactive thymidine. It was a vast library containing stories of the wiring of the brain. Owing to eventual radioactive decay, the pages of this library would one day be blank. Professor Rakic graciously offered the use of his slides so that we might discover new developmental pathways in the brain. Fixated on Reissner's fiber, which, not being a cell, was unlabeled, I declined the offer.

About the time I had begun my search for the anatomical basis of *kundalini* yoga, I wrote to Sir John Eccles who had won the Nobel Prize for his work on the synapse. I was attracted to his belief that the soul is not reducible to the physical brain. I had hoped that he would be sympathetic to my quest and might add to my knowledge of the neurophysiology of the central canal. He replied with a gracious supportive letter saying that his book *Facing Reality: Philosophical Adventures of a Brain Scientist* was consistent with my philosophical outlook.

Shortly after my discovery of Reissner's fiber, I again wrote to Eccles to tell of that discovery. "I am alarmed that you have identified the primitive symbols of yoga with actual anatomical structures!" he replied.

Five years later, as the presenter of the influential and prestigious 1978 Gifford Lectures, established in 1887 "to promote and diffuse the study of natural theology in the widest sense of the term—in other words the knowledge of God," Eccles said:

> I accept all of the discoveries and well-corroborated hypotheses of science—not as absolute truth, but as the nearest approach to truth that has yet been attained. But these lectures will reveal in case after case that here is an important residue not explained by science, and even beyond any future explanation by science. This leads on to the theme of Natural Theology with the idea of a Supernatural beyond the explanatory power of science ... As a dualist, I believe in the reality of the world of mind or spirit as well as in the reality of the material world. Furthermore, I am a finalist in the sense of believing that there is some Design in the process of biological evolution that has eventually led to us self-conscious beings with our unique individuality ... I will suggest in later lectures that we are creatures with some supernatural meaning as yet ill-defined.

A few weeks after Dr. Loeser's phone call, I arrived at Woods Hole, a tiny village by the sea. Every year, this close-knit community of local fishermen and shopkeepers prepared for the summer's onslaught of tourists, shoppers, and visiting scientists with a huge banner reading, *Tourists Go Home!* The National Marine Fishery Lab, known as the Woods Hole Laboratory of the United States Fish Commission from 1895 to 1958, no longer conducted basic research. Nevertheless, salt water in the two large circular stone tanks still circulated, and the cabinets, furniture, and scarred lab bench remained. As I unpacked my dissecting kit, preparing to learn Porter Sargent's surgical procedure to expose the fiber, a curious coincidence sent a shiver down my spine. Reading the acknowledgments of Sargent's paper, I learned that I was sitting at the very same lab bench on which he had sat seventy years earlier!

After several failures, I peeled away the membrane covering the fourth ventricle of a sedated shark. I gently inserted the curved needle probe into the cavity, and, sensing a slight pressure, slowly lifted the probe. Reissner's fiber briefly sparkled beneath the light of a 100-watt bulb reflecting from the rolled rim parabola-shaped reflector of an antique flexible brass gooseneck desk lamp. Then it slithered off the hook into the bloodied pool below.

Excited to share the good news with Dr. Loeser, and eager to plan the next steps—finding a suitable animal that could interface with Dr. Loeser's instrument—I wrote him a letter. Several days later, I received a frantic phone call from my parents. The Dean had called our home, looking for me. The administration didn't know where I was. Dr. Loesers' melanoma had rapidly metastasized. He was dead.

Immediately I realized what had happened. Dr. Loeser knew that because classes were optional, my absence would go unnoticed. Exams were graded anonymously using a student code. Only a failed or missed exam would bring a student to the attention of the faculty. For several months his plan had worked. He knew that soon he would no longer be able to protect my dreams. He wanted to give me time to nourish them so that they would be strong enough to survive the onslaught that was sure to follow.

Because I had paid the tuition, and because Dr. Loeser had arranged for me to receive $400 for an Independent Student Research Project, I was deemed eligible to receive credit for my research, contingent on passing the required thesis. However, the dentist who was in charge of the Thesis Committee took exception to my "Speculative Quantum Biophysical Model of Kundalini Yoga." "Fanciful gibberish! Travesty of a research project!" he scrawled on the cover. When I asked if he could be more specific, he screamed, "We don't care what you think! Tell us exactly what you did and what you observed." So my revised medical student research thesis describing my surgical procedures and my observations now sits on the shelves of the Lyman Maynard Stowe Library of the UCONN Health Center along with hundreds of other unread theses.

The Devil had won another battle to keep the fiber in oblivion.

Seven

Is the Old Testament an Account of the Breakdown of the Bicameral Mind?

Introduction

According to Jaynes, the actors and authors of the Old Testament were originally nonconscious individuals organized into a hierarchical theocracy governed by hallucinatory gods. About 3,000 years ago, this bicameral system broke down when those individuals became refugees from war torn countries. This breakdown resulted in a turbulent, violent transition from bicamerality to subjective consciousness. The validity of Jaynes's interpretation of the Old Testament requires evidence of bicameral sources, an account of its chaotic breakdown consistent with the Biblical text, and an explanation of the persistence of the beliefs from the supposed lost bicameral era. Jaynes fails to support all three pillars of his interpretation.

Bicameral Origins of the Old Testament?

Relying primarily on the *Encyclopedia Britannica* in "matters of dating, authorship, and other exegetical material on the Old Testament," Jaynes aligned himself with the documentary hypothesis that the Old Testament began as a "pious fraud," which, in Jaynes's words, were "forgeries of the seventh, sixth and fifth centuries BC, brilliant workings of brightly colored strands from a scatter of places and periods." It all began with the "discovery" of Deuteronomy by King Josiah in 621 BC in the First Temple in Jerusalem. The first problem confronting Jaynes's interpretation is his attempt to attribute the originals of the "forgeries" to bicameral sources.

Jaynes cites Amos from the eighth century BC as the oldest "pure" book written by a bicameral author. However, if we remove the filters of the bicameral mind, which creates the mirage of Biblical prophets as nonconscious individuals governed by command auditory hallucinations, we find that Amos was a fully conscious individual admonishing his fellow Israelites to follow God's laws, to love good and work for social justice.

"Amos never ponders anything in his heart; he can't; he would not know what it meant," declares Jaynes. Yet Amos passionately preached about social justice in language that continues to reach our hearts. Martin Luther King, in his "I Have a Dream Speech," quoted Amos's prayer: "But let justice roll on like a river, righteousness like a never-failing stream!" If metaphorical language is the stuff of consciousness, then Amos was fully conscious. Also, Amos preached against the performance of rituals that could be carried out by bicameral automatons. He preached that empty ritual is unworthy in the eyes of the Lord. He preached that God demanded love and justice, a demand that requires recognition of the inner life of oneself and of others.

Jaynes notes that on the few occasions that Amos speaks of himself, he is abrupt, declaring that he is no prophet, but a "gatherer of sycamore fruit." According to Jaynes Amos "does not consciously think before he speaks; in fact he does not think as we do at all: his thought is done for him." However, Amos's declaration that he is no prophet, but gatherer of sycamore fruit was a deliberate reply to Amaziah's insinuation that Amos was a mercenary prophet who deceived others for personal gain. Amos did not earn his "bread" by prophesizing. He was called by the Lord. Amos clearly understood deceit, a hallmark of Jaynesian consciousness.

Having dubiously cited Amos as an extreme example of bicamerality, Jaynes suggests that Ecclesiastes is an example of subjective consciousness from the second century BC. This is problematic for a variety of reasons. First, 180 BC is the latest possible date of the writing of Ecclesiastes because the Jewish writer Ben Sira quotes from it then. While tradition attributes the writing of Ecclesiastes to King Solomon during the tenth century BC, it is clear that it has been edited. Most scholarly analyses of its language, style, and possible cultural influences suggest that it was written during the fifth century BC. However, there is strong evidence to suggest that King Solomon himself is the primary source of Ecclesiastes. I Kings, written during the sixth century BC, declares, "King Solomon was greater in riches and wisdom than all the other kings of the earth. The whole world sought audience with Solomon to hear the wisdom God had put in his heart" (I Kings 10:23-24). The Talmud says, "Hezekiah (720-692 BC) and his assistants recorded Isaiah, Proverbs, Song of Songs and Ecclesiastes" (b. B. Bathra 15a). Proverbs 25:1 says, "These are the proverbs of Solomon which the men of Hezekiah, king of Judah, transcribed." These passages can only mean that some written record or oral tradition pre-existed Hezekiah. Further evidence that the writing dates to the monarchic period is the advice given: keep the king's commands (8:2), curse not the king (10:20), and woe to thee when the king was a boy (10:2). This advice would be irrelevant after the monarchic period.

To further his case that Ecclesiastes is the work of subjective consciousness divorced from bicamerality, Jaynes contends, "god is rarely mentioned." However, Ecclesiastes 5:1–7 taught that one should listen carefully to God and faithfully follow one's vows to Him:

> Guard your steps when you go to the house of God. Go near to listen rather than to offer the sacrifice of fools, who do not know that they do wrong. Do not be quick with your mouth, do not be hasty in your heart to utter anything before God. God is in heaven and you are on earth, so let your words be few. A dream comes when there are many cares, and many words mark the speech of a fool. When you make a vow to God, do not delay to fulfill it. He has no pleasure in fools; fulfill your vow.

Ecclesiastes concludes: "Let us hear the conclusion of the whole matter: Fear God, and keep his commandments: for this is the whole duty of man" (Ecclesiastes 12:13).

While it is true, as Jaynes points out, that some scholars believe that references to God are later interpolations, the history of Solomon as recorded in I Kings and the Books of Chronicles describe an individual who sought God's guidance. In conclusion, the evidence suggests that Amos was a fully conscious individual who claimed to have received the gift of prophecy. Ecclesiastes does not represent a stark constrict to Amos either in the date of its composition or in the author's professed allegiance to God. Amos was indeed more passionate about his prophetic experiences than Solomon was. But this passion was not a product of overactive hallucinatory neural circuits, but rather a reflection of the times. Amos was pleading with his people to follow the Lord before their disobedience brought the destruction of Jerusalem. Solomon reigned during a period of unparalleled prosperity and stability organized around worship of the Lord in the Temple he had built.

According to Jaynes, the story of the Fall is a myth of the breakdown of the bicameral mind and origin of consciousness. The problems of interpreting the story of the Fall as the coming of consciousness "should," he believes, "be rationalistically contrasted with the Odyssey" because "both raise the question of how nonconscious bicameral individuals narrated their coming to consciousness." Such a rational contrast confronts two problems for Jaynes's interpretation.

First, Jaynes contends that the bicameral mind of the Hebrews started to break down during the end of the second millennium BC. However, the extremely detailed genealogy from Adam and Eve, to Cain, Enoch, Methuselah, Noah, Abraham, Isaac, Jacob, Moses, and King David places the story in the sixth millennium BC. Second, unlike the *Odyssey*, which supposedly developed through an evolution of "pre-conscious hypostases," starting with nonconscious automatons of the *Iliad*, the story of the Fall has no prequel. It is a story of Creation. According to Genesis, the cunning serpent spoke to Eve on the afternoon she was created.

Jaynes's belief that the story of Jacob dates to before 1000 BC is inconsistent with his hypothesis that Jacob possessed a nonconscious bicameral mentality. The story of Jacob describes conscious individuals practiced in the art of deception: Jacob deceived his father Isaac to gain his brother's birthright, and his father-in-law, Laban, deceived him into marrying Leah. No reasonable interpretation of Genesis would place the story of the Fall after the story of Jacob. Also, twice Abraham, Jacob's grandfather, passes Sarah off as his sister (Genesis 12:10–20, 20:1–18) and Isaac, Abraham's son, passes off Rebekah as his sister (Genesis 26:16).

Were the Hebrews Khabirus?

Jaynes's contention that the Old Testament originated from the stories and writings of an amorphous mass of refugees and outcasts known as khabiru is inconsistent with historical facts. The Babylonian and the similar sounding Egyptian word were used pejoratively to describe paupers, robbers, slaves, or mercenaries. The term does not refer an ethnic group but to a social class. There is neither a linguistic connection between *khabiru* and *ivrit*, the Hebrew word for "Hebrew," nor a connection between the khabiru and the Hebrews. That the Hebrews have been an ethnic group united by language, culture, history, and religion for more than 3,000 years is attested by several converging lines of evidence.

Indeed, Jaynes's dating of the beginning of the "story or the imagined story of the later Khabiru or Hebrews" to Josiah's discovery of scrolls in the Temple of Jerusalem in 621 BC supports the identity of the Hebrews as distinct from the khabirus. Why would there be a temple dedicated to the worship of the God of Israel if the Hebrews were an amorphous mass of vagrants?

Further supporting the distinct ethnicity of the Hebrews are 1) the Merneptah Stele which bears an inscription referring to King Merneptah's victory over Israel between 1213 to 1203 BC, 2) the Mesha

Stele from 840 BC which contains a lengthy description of how King Mesha of Moab overcame its subjugation to Israel, 3) the Kurkh Monoliths, two Assyrian stelae that refer to Ahab, King of Israel, and 4) the recently (1994) discovered Tel Dan Stele which describe Hazael's victory over the king of Israel and his ally the king from the "House of David." Also, analysis of the mutation rate of genetic markers of Jews who currently identify themselves as Cohanim showed they originated from a common ancestor about 3,300 years ago. This is consistent with the timeline predicted by the traditional belief that Cohanim are descendants of Moses' brother Aaron.

Jaynes's interpretation of Genesis 47:18-26 as evidence of Hebrews "in the desperation of hunger, bartering control of their lives for bread and seed," is contrary to the meaning of the text. Genesis 47 tells the story of how Abraham's great grandson Joseph rose to become the second most powerful leader of Egypt. He advised the Pharaoh to store grain during times of famine and, as a result, the Pharaoh greatly extended his power over the Egyptians. Joseph's brothers and their families then joined him in Egypt and during the following 300 hundred years the Hebrew population grew. Subsequent rulers of Egypt, fearing the Hebrews' potential as adversaries, enslaved them. Moses then liberated the enslaved Hebrews.

"Yahweh"

Jaynes's contention that the creation story was rewritten by a group of khabiru between the seventh and fifth centuries BC, who were following only Yahweh and wanted to make him warmer and more human, is contradicted by the text and the evidence of history. According to Jaynes, *elohim* is incorrectly translated as God. It is plural and, although it takes a singular verb, actually refers to the multitude of hallucinatory voices that the ancient khabirus followed as gods. Yahweh was the voice followed by a particular group of khabiru. Jaynes claims that most scholars dismiss the translation found in most Bibles—"I AM THAT I AM"—as folk etymology akin to claiming that the derivation of Manhattan comes from a man on the island with a hat on.

However, nearly two millennia of theological analysis and tradition from Talmudic sages, to medieval scholars, to current theologians, and Hebrew grammar, contradict Jaynes's interpretations. The translation of Yahweh as "I AM THAT I AM" comes from Exodus 3:14 when God tells Moses, "Ehyeh asher Ehyeh." Ehyeh is the first person singular imperfect of the verb "haya," to be. "Asher" is a pronoun that can mean "who," "that," "which," or "where." "I AM THAT I AM" closely follows the Hebrew. Yahweh is the German transliteration of the Tetragrammaton, the four Hebrew letters of God's name, which is unutterable, except by the holiest Temple priest. It represents the infinite, transcendent, personal essence of God. *Elohim* represents the cosmic manifestations and the divine justice that emanate from His essence. Yahweh is transcendent. He encompasses, and permeates, the immanent. He is the eternal one who encompasses and permeates the temporal.

Jaynes's assertion that the Old Testament reflects polytheism based on a multitude of hallucinatory voices not only defies thousands of years of theology, but relies on a uniquely idiosyncratic translation of Psalm 42 that replaces the universally accepted translation of the Psalm as David's longing for God with:

> As the stag pants after the waterbrooks,
> So pants my mind after you, O gods!
> My mind thirsts for gods! for living gods!
> When shall I come face to face with gods?

The Ebla tablets discovered in 1974 suggest that the idea of a transcendent God who created and rules heaven and earth, and of prophets who announced His message, developed from a stable culture that was an important source of Hebrew culture. Ebla began as small community in Syria around 3500 BC and developed into a flourishing city with about 30,000 inhabitants by 2500. The Ebla tablets consist of 20,000 cuneiform tablets written in a proto-Canaanite and proto-Hebraic language.

Based on a philological analysis, Professor Paolo Matthaie, head of the project, declared: "The Ebla tablets establish the patriarchs and their names as historical realities." And, "We have found the civilization that was the background of the people of the Old Testament."

The renowned paleographer Giovanni Pettinato, a specialist in Elbaic language who continued research on the tablets, translated a creation story inscribed on the tablets:

> Lord of Heaven and earth:
> The earth was not, you created it,
> The light of day was not, you created it,
> The morning light you had not [yet] made exist.

Pettinato showed that the universal term Lord represented a new concept of God as an "abstract entity." God is seen as a transcendent being who created and rules the cosmos but "is continually present upon the earth and in daily life." The Elbaic language shows a progression toward the use of term "Ya" to designate the Lord during the reign of

King Ebrum around 2500 BC. Like the Tetragrammaton that transliterates as Yahweh, "Ya" was not to be pronounced. While the resemblance between "Ya" and Yahweh, and between Ebrum and Abram, the name that was changed by God to Abraham, might be coincidental, there is clear evidence of prophets who spread the world of the Lord.

"But the most pleasant surprise," wrote Pettinato, "is finding attested in this early period holy men not bound to the worship of a particular god but rather representing a new type of religiosity. These are the 'prophets' belonging to the category of prophesiers of the divine word. These holy men, specified by the country of origin, moved from one city to another announcing the divine message."

Regardless of the connection between "Ya" and "Yahweh," and regardless of whether either or both were hallucinations or mystical experiences of God, it is clear that the creation story of Yahweh was not rewritten to make Yahweh warmer and more human. After Adam and Eve ate from the forbidden fruit of the Tree of Knowledge Yahweh-Elohim said to the woman: "I will make your pains in childbearing very severe; with painful labor you will give birth to children. Your desire will be for your husband, and he will rule over you."

To Adam he said, "Because you listened to your wife and ate fruit from the tree about which I commanded you, 'You must not eat from it.' Cursed is the ground because of you; through painful toil you will eat food from it all the days of your life. It will produce thorns and thistles for you, and you will eat the plants of the field. By the sweat of your brow you will eat your food until you return to the ground, since from it you were taken; for dust you are and to dust you will return" (Genesis 3:16–19). And Yahweh-Elohim banished him from the Garden of Eden (Genesis 3:23). The introduction of pain, suffering toil, and death by "Yahweh" hardly served the purpose of making of enhancing his humanity.

Is the Old Testament the Story of the Breakdown of the Bicameral Mind?

Even if one accepts, in defiance of reason and without textual evidence, that the Old Testament originated from a bicameral era, the contention that the Old Testament tells the story of the breakdown of the bicameral mind is inconsistent with the clear meaning of the text.

Jaynes contends that Moses was a witness to the early stages of the breakdown of the bicameral mind, the loss of its visual component. Reading the text of Genesis literally and relying on the hypothesis that all Biblical references to God are actually references to hallucinations,

Jaynes writes that during the "true bicameral period, there was a visual component to the hallucinated voice." He cites Adam and Eve hearing God walking in the garden, shutting the door of Noah's Ark, and appearing before Abraham at Sichem, Bethel, and Hebron as evidence of visual hallucinations. He compares Jacob's wrestling with God to scuffling all night with a hoodlum. That these events represent visionary experiences rather than hallucinatory experiences is not considered by Jaynes.

According to Jaynes, the visual component of Moses' bicamerality reflected its breakdown. God appeared to Moses as "a burning bush, a cloud, a huge pillar of fire." God proclaims to Moses, "You cannot see My face, for no man can see Me and live!" (Exodus 33:20). As the visual component of the bicameral mind changed, the hallucinatory voice of Yahweh became unstable. When the Hebrews were in "precarious pursuit of some hallucinated vision," the last of the vanishing remnant of the hallucinatory gods was "as petty and foot-stompingly petulant as any human tyrant under questioning." However, astonishingly, the "greatest teaching of the entire Old Testament" was revealed: Yahweh "becomes something written upon tablets, he becomes law, something unchanging, approachable by all, something relatable to all men equally, king and shepherd, universal and transcendent." But, how could the last decompensating psychotic hallucinatory voice become the written law that reflects something transcendent and universal, something that became the numinous core of the Abrahamic religions? Of all the implausible feats Jaynes attributes to the bicameral mind, from building the ziggurats and pyramids to writing the *Iliad* to governing a hierarchical theocracy, its authorship of universal laws reflecting the will of a transcendent God, laws that have dominated Western civilization, is the most implausible.

If, for the sake of argument, the Old Testament *is* an account of the breakdown of the bicameral mind and the birth pangs of consciousness, would nostalgia for the authority of lost hallucinatory gods have provided the basis for religion? Nostalgia implies conscious recollection of memories. The nonconscious automatons of the bicameral era who were commanded by auditory hallucinations would not have formed consciousness memories. If we allow for "unconscious nostalgia"—memories stored and transmitted by a collective unconscious—then we are confronted with the problem that such memories must have overcome the conscious recorded memories of psychotic decompensation, mockery, persecution, and eventual extermination of bicameral individuals.

Nonconscious Hallucinating Prophets, True Prophets, and False Prophets

For Jaynes, all Biblical prophecy was the vocalization of auditory hallucinations without conscious volition or cognition. There was neither true prophecy, which requires communication with God and therefore entails a "metaphysical imposition," nor false prophecy, which requires deceit and therefore entails consciousness. This omission of both true and false prophets disregards the crucial distinction that underlies the Biblical account of prophecy.

The first example of Jaynes's disregard of the distinction between true and false prophets is his telling of the "discovery" of Deuteronomy by King Josiah in 621 BC in the First Temple in Jerusalem. According to Jaynes, the manuscript of Deuteronomy was discovered *after* Josiah had "ordered the temple cleaned and cleared of its remaining bicameral rites." However, this assertion contradicts the story of Josiah as told in the Old Testament. In II Kings, the story is told how the royal scribe Shaphan read the dire prophecies from Deuteronomy regarding the terrible fate that would befall the people for forsaking God and worshipping strange gods, Josiah rent his clothes and sent a delegation led by the High Priest to seek out the prophet Jeremiah. Because Jeremiah was not in Judah at the time, the king's delegation consulted the prophetess Huldah. She sent word to the King because he had humbled himself before God, he would not witness the devastation of the Temple. It was only *after* having read from Deuteronomy that Josiah instituted the reforms and cleansed the Temple of idols.

The reforms instituted by Josiah could not have been a cleansing of the remaining bicameral rites. Otherwise, Josiah would not have consulted a prophetess to guide his actions. The worship of Yahweh would have been among the bicameral rites that Jaynes contends Josiah was cleansing. Josiah directed the elimination of idols, false priests, and the worship of pagan gods, but rededicated himself to worshipping Yahweh. If Josiah's justification for cleansing the remaining bicameral rites from the Temple had been Deuteronomy, it would not have proclaimed the unity of *elohim* and "Yahweh": "Hear O Israel, the Lord ("Yahweh") is our God (*elohim*) the Lord is one." Why would, Deuteronomy proclaim the unity of Yahweh and *Elohim* if its purpose was a subterfuge to eliminate all the *elohim* other than Yahweh?

According to Jaynes, I Kings describes events from the eleventh century BC that reflect the psychology of the eighth century BC and were put into writing about one hundred years after Josiah discovered the manuscript of Deuteronomy. It is, according to Jaynes, an account of the breakdown of the bicameral mind. Indeed, Jaynes writes,

"Bicamerality, in a rather decadent form is represented in the wild gangs of nabiim, the winnowed chaff of the Khabiru ... roaming outside the cities in the hills, speaking the voices they hear within themselves but believe to come from outside them, answering the voices using music and drums to increase their excitement." This shattered bicamerality ultimately descended into the horrors of psychotic decompensation, persecution, and genocidal extermination until the last Hebrew prophets during Babylonian exile during the fifth century BC.

Jaynes's misreading of the Old Testament's description of the treatment of prophets is illustrated in the following examples. According to Jaynes, in 835 BC Ahab and Jahoshaphat rounded up 400 prophets like cattle to hear their hue and clamor and later, hundreds herded up, they were raving and copying each other like schizophrenics in a back ward. However, according to the Bible, Ahab was seduced by his nefarious wife Jezebel into worshipping idols and persecuting true prophets. During the encounter between Ahab and Jahoshaphat, the righteous King Jahoshaphat insisted that a true prophet of the Lord be consulted before heeding advice of Ahab's prophets who were proclaiming that Ahab would emerge victorious over Ramoth Gilead. Ahab said that Micaiah was a true prophet of the Lord, but he objected to seeking his council because he never prophesized anything good about the king. Nevertheless, heeding Jahoshaphat's advice, Micaiah was summoned. He prophesized that Ahab's armies would be defeated and that he would be killed. Ahab imprisoned Micaiah and shortly thereafter died in battle.

Jaynes's citing of I Kings 18:4 as evidence that the last remnants of bicameral communities "were hunted down and exterminated like wild animals" also contradicts the text. Obadiah hid 100 prophets in caves to save them from Jezebel's murder of the true prophets. He was blessed with the gift of prophecy for his heroism.

Jaynes refers to the Biblical account of the prophecies of Hananiah and Jeremiah as the "somewhat ridiculous competition between Hananiah and Jeremiah as to whose bicameral voice is the right one." However, the Book of Jeremiah clearly portrays Jeremiah as a true prophet and Hananiah as a false one. Jeremiah prophesized that as result of their turning away from God the Jews must temporarily subject themselves to the yoke of the Babylonians and surrender to their king. He therefore urged the King of Judea, Zedekiah, who was placed on the throne by the Babylonian King, Nebuchadnezzar, after he had besieged Jerusalem and deposed Zedeliah's uncle, King Josiah, not to form military alliances to defeat King Nebuchadnezzar. Jeremiah also prophesized that the Jews would return to Jerusalem after a seventy-year exile. Hananiah, telling the people what they wanted hear, falsely prophesized that the Jewish army would be victorious and overthrow the Babylonians.

According to Jaynes, it was only the death of Hananiah two months after his dispute with Jeremiah that prevented the Old Testament from including the Book of Hananiah instead of the Book of Jeremiah. However, even if Hananiah had outlived Jeremiah, there would not have been a Book of Hananiah. Zedekiah's refusal to surrender to King Nebuchadnezzar resulted in the killings of his sons in front of him, the very last thing he saw before he was blinded. The people's homes, the King's palaces, and the Temple in Jerusalem were destroyed. After a seventy-year exile, the Jews returned to Jerusalem and rebuilt the Temple. Hananiah was judged to be a false prophet. Jeremiah was judged to be a true prophet.

Jaynes cited Zechariah 13:3, "And if anyone still prophesies, then his father and mother who gave birth to him will say to him, 'You shall not live, for you have spoken falsely in the name of the LORD'; and his father and mother who gave birth to him will pierce him through when he prophesies," as evidence that sixth-century BC prophets were calling for the extermination of all prophets to "move the gene pool toward subjectivity." However, he ignores Zechariah's words that anyone who prophesized at that time would have spoken falsely in the name of the Lord.

Conclusion

Jaynes's argument that the Old Testament is an account of the breakdown of the bicameral mind and that religion is nostalgia for lost hallucinatory gods — even if one accepts the reality of the bicameral mind — is unsubstantiated. However, his belief that the Old Testament is based on a state of consciousness radically different from our own inspires us to explore new neuropsychological interpretations of religion.

Jaynes rejects the idea that the prophets communicated with the eternal, infinite God who created and rules the universe. Such revelatory experiences, for Jaynes, would have constituted a "metaphysical imposition" like the ones that had expelled Wallace from the scientific community. However, neurocosmological models of Reissner's fiber could provide a scientific basis for supersensory knowledge of the Absolute. Religion might be reverence for the memories of the collective revelation at Mt. Sinai, and the personal revelations of Old Testament prophets, Jesus and Mohammed. Reinforcing that reverence would be perinatal imprinting of our neural circuits by Reissner's fiber.

Eight

The Legacy of Julian Jaynes
Shining New Light Through the Cracks of the Bicameral Mind

Julian Jaynes's magnificent failure to explain the origin of consciousness challenges us to re-examine a fundamental tenet of the current neuroscientific paradigm: consciousness has evolved slowly, steadily, and continuously. As Jaynes points out, the marvelous continuity of life, that Darwin and other naturalists have discovered, blinds us to the "terrifying and absolute" discontinuity of human consciousness. Whereas our simian ancestors have repeated genetically programmed patterns of behavior for millions of years, humans have liberated themselves from stimulus bound, programmed behavior to contemplate their origin and change their destiny. In the short span of 6,000 years, we have created a world of knowledge that has taken us from fire to atomic energy, from the wheel to spaceships, from marks on stone to electronic terabytes, and from the natural selection of random variations to genetic engineering. Mathematical models of reality verified with technological marvels point toward supersensible, transtemporal realties. Only humans have created what Karl Popper called the world of objective knowledge, what Teilhard de Chardin called the noosphere, and what is known to kabbalists as *Da'at*.

Jaynes also compels us to re-examine our assumptions about the earliest religious texts. They are not merely primitive superstitions and myths. They also contain factual accounts based on states of consciousness radically different from our own. They provide windows into the recent launching of human consciousness on its vertical trajectory.

Exploring Jaynes's hypothesis that schizophrenia is, at least in part, a return to the mentality of the Old Testament prophets could lead to a new understanding of the neuropsychological origins of religion and the etiology of schizophrenia. Having worked intensively with schizophrenics during my early career as a psychiatrist, I can attest to the fascinating intersection between genuine religious experiences and psychosis. During the prodromal and acute psychotic phase of their illness, many schizophrenics report numinous encounters. While auditory hallucinations typically do not dominate these experiences, they are a core feature of schizophrenia, and God "spoke" to the prophets.

Jaynes's hypothesis that schizophrenics are vestiges from the era of prophecy when prophets interpreted command auditory hallucinations issued from the right temporal lobe as the voices of the "gods" is consistent with neuroimaging studies of hallucinating schizophrenics. The hypothesis that schizophrenia is a vestige of an era of prophecy neurologically based on Reissner's fiber is consistent with research conducted by Grigory Vilkov. He injected serum from schizophrenics into rats and showed it had significant neurotropic effects on the subcommissural organ, and it impaired aldosterone production by the adrenal cortex, which is regulated by the subcommissural organ. Because the average age of onset for schizophrenia in men is 18 and 25 for women, the presence of antibodies against the source of Reissner's fiber in the serum of schizophrenics suggests the persistence of the fiber well past its typical perinatal involution. Individuals with "physio-kundalini syndrome" or "Qi-gong Psychotic reaction," diagnostic categories on the fringes of the Diagnostic and Statistical Manual describing a possible overlap of psychopathology and genuine *kundalini* or *Qi* awakening, could also provide attractive subjects for an investigation of the possibility that they are vestiges from the era of the origin of mystical traditions. The answer to the crucial question of whether the experiences associated with either the right temporal lobe or Reissner's fiber are hallucinations or encounters with the "Eternal, Infinite, Absolute Good" about Whom Reverent Jaynes preached lies in the unexplored realm of neurocosmology.

An unintended part of Jaynes's legacy is that our misgivings about his preposterous proposition that consciousness arose from hallucinating members of advanced civilizations who were actually noncomscious physical systems reacting to their environments compels us to reassess the foundation of neuroscience: consciousness emerged from the evolution of matter. Perhaps the perennial intuition that consciousness is prior to matter, trampled upon by Darwinism, is true. Another unintended part of Jaynes's legacy is that his factual interpretation of our earliest religious texts brings attention to the possibility that the earliest references to God were not descriptions of hallucinations but descriptions of the consciousness of the consciousness behind natural laws and the supersensory perceptions of transcendent realities.

Inspired by Jaynes's recognition of humankind's evolutionarily recent leap of consciousness and his factual interpretation of religious texts, and the implications of his failures, I propose a unified neurocosmology organized around Reissner's fiber based on the following conjectures:

I. The infinite regress of the consciousness of consciousness, free will, and the human capacity to discover natural laws and mathematical truths imply that consciousness is infinite and eternal.

II. Descriptions of the "subtle anatomy," the purported anatomical connection between human consciousness and the Absolute described by our earliest mystical traditions, were based on interoceptions of Reissner's fiber.

III. Extrapolating backward in time, we encounter the initial singularity, a transcendent fusion of nothingness and infinity, the zero-point energy of the "quantum foam" that pre-exists space and time. It invisibly permeates our being. It is the cosmic intelligence behind natural laws and the basis their physical manifestation. It is the stuff of consciousness.

IV. Direct consciousness of macroscopic quantum systems achieved by Reissner's fiber could open the doors of perception to realities currently inaccessible to our phenomenal awareness and which currently are tenuously grasped by mathematics.

Contemplation of the origin of spacetime from the pregeometric, transtemporal initial singularity brings us to the limits of understanding. And, is time itself an illusion? Einstein once wrote, "Isn't philosophy all written in honey? It seems clear to one at first; afterward it's all gone, only the pap remains." Heeding his warning, we will build our speculations on the tangible foundation of Reissner's fiber.

Five hundred millions years ago, during the Cambrian explosion, as the global architecture of the hollow brain was established by the first protovertebrates, glycoproteins secreted into the fluid-filled central cavities aggregated around a one-dimensional thread to form Reissner's fiber. This macroscopic structure greatly amplified quantum coherences achieved by similar microscopic structures such as the microtubules constituting cilia, centrioles, mitotic spindles, neuronal cytoskeletons, etc. The relationship between consciousness and physical reality was thereby greatly strengthened.

Sentient vertebrates began to roam the earth and evolved into *Homo sapiens* 200,000 years ago. One hundred thousand years ago, during the commission of the metaphysical original sin and the creation of the digital infinity of language, epigenetic factors caused the typical perinatal involution of the fiber in humans. Human consciousness liberated itself from stimulus bound reactivity. An abyss now separated human consciousness from its eternal source. The fiber's persistence as a morphogenetic structure during human embryonic development helped to wire the billions of neurons and trillions of synapses that interact with quantum biophysical events and initiate the classical activities of neural spikes and muscle contractions that provide the basis for speech and action.

Six thousand years ago the digital infinity of language converged upon its center in a few rare individuals in China, India, and Mesopotamia, for whom Reissner's fiber persisted into adulthood. Their consciousness transiently experienced its lost connection to its eternal creator. These geniuses transcended themselves. Their leap of consciousness was commensurate with the transilience from "nothing" to "something," from the pregeometric, transtemporal initial singularity to spacetime. Chinese, Indian, and Hebrew mystics, respectively, named this ineffable convergence the *Tao, Brahman,* and the *Ein-Sof,* from which the unity of the cosmic infinitude of *Elohim* and the Infinite personal God represented by the ineffable Tetragrammaton transliterated as Yahweh derives. Seeking atonement for the metaphysical original sin, they tried to grasp interoceptions of Reissner's fiber with the digital infinity of language. They struggled to grasp their experiences with the finite, self-referential web of language wherein every thought becomes its opposite. They committed the Biblical original sin by creating self-contained systems to reflect good or evil, truth or falsity. They chose to govern themselves by them. Thus, they decoupled themselves from natural laws and followed conflicting ideologies and versions of the truth. They were exiled from Paradise. But descriptions of Reissner's fiber provided a physical basis for neurocosmological atonement.

There was no returning to Paradise through the gate from which they had left. There was no returning to the passive, dream harmony of humanity, God, and the universe after the active imagination and intellect had experienced the Infinite. Cherubim and a flaming sword flashing back and forth now guarded the Eastern gate back to Reissner's fiber, the Tree of Life. But the stroboscopic flash of Reissner's fiber's imprint on the primitive, kaleidoscopic web of knowledge remained as they began their 7,000-year journey to the Western gate of Eden searching for the infinite with the seemingly finite flesh.

As the last transient, partial flashes of Reissner's fiber faded into oblivion, and prophecy ended during Axial Age, humankind's journey along the road of science began. Thales and Pythagoras led the way in ancient Greece during the sixth century BC.

According to Jaynes, science's quest for unity and certainty, for evidence of God's handiwork in Nature, is rooted in nostalgia for lost hallucinatory gods. Science's misguided faith that it could know the mind of God has led to atheism and quasi-religious scientisms. But, as we stand before science's current impasses—quantum uncertainty, incompatibilities between general relativity and quantum mechanics, mathematical undecidability, and mysteries about the origin of life and the relationship between mind and matter—another possibility appears before us. Science's journey has not been driven by nostalgia for lost hallucinatory gods produced by naturally selected random variations of matter, but by the "rapturous amazement at the harmony of natural law, which reveals an intelligence of such superiority that, compared with it, all the systematic thinking and acting of human beings is utterly insignificant reflection." Which is the basis of Einstein's cosmic religion.

Perhaps, beyond our rapturous amazement there are lost secrets about the consciousness of a meter-long, one-dimensional transtemporal thread ensheathed by quantum coherent 5-nanometer filaments comprising Reissner's fiber. This lost consciousness was transmitted orally for thousands of years. It is imprinted perinatally in the personal unconscious. Its ultimate unity eludes language. As we follow the ineffable *Tao*, *Brahman*, and *Ein-Sof* from the center of the self-referential web of language their meanings transform into opposites. These opposites are not contradictions or complementary pairs but elements of a higher unity. Ultimately, when interoceptions of Reissner's fiber are fully integrated with exteroceptions at the limits of objectivity, science will fall away like Wittgenstein's ladder and the Mystical will show itself.

The earliest theologians and philosophers recognized that God is beyond the grasp of the intellect. But our free will operating within the range of quantum uncertainty in the microstructures of the brain can create knowledge that allows us to participate in the unfolding of God's eternal consciousness. Not only are we not mere "helpless spectators" but we are cocreators of a new heaven and a new earth.

The Road Forward

The road toward exploring the final frontiers of the possible role of Reissner's fiber in human consciousness is long. The first challenge along the road is that, with possible rare exceptions, the fiber is not present in the adult human brain. The subcommissural organ, the primary source of the fiber, typically starts to atrophy by the fifth month of fetal development and becomes vestigial by the fourth year of childhood. The central canal is occluded in the majority of adults. The terminal ventricle at the end of the central canal typically atrophies by the age of forty. Nevertheless, the genetic machinery necessary for producing Reissner's fiber exists in humans and there are marked variations in its expression. A fully developed subcommissural organ has been observed in a 60-year-old man. Neither the occlusion of the central canal nor the atrophy of the terminal ventricle is universal. Reissner's fiber was observed in a 14-year-old.

The first step toward exploring the role of Reissner's fiber in human consciousness would be to regenerate the fiber and its associated structures. This could be achieved by reversing the epigenetic factors that limit the expression of genes responsible for the production of the fiber. Pharmacological agents could also enhance secretion of components of the fiber into the ventricles. Because the subcommissural organ is outside the blood brain barrier, exogenous components could be introduced.

In addition to developing the mechanisms needed to produce the fiber, one would also need to ensure that the passageways through which the fiber travels are patent. Exercises similar to the rhythmic breathing, breath-holding, muscular locks, stretches, and postures of yoga could straighten the canal and direct pressurized waves of CSF through it. Currently available imaging devices could monitor progress.

Subjective reports of interoceptions consistent with the presence of the fiber would provide supporting evidence of the presence of the fiber. However, such perceptions might be generated by alterations of CSF dynamics or chemistry rather than the fiber itself. Current imaging devices lack the resolution and sensitivity to create images of Reissner's fiber. However, new technologies, perhaps based on nanoprobes such as quantum dots or nitrogen vacancy diamonds, offer the hope of measuring the fiber's activities.

Alternatively, searches for individuals who have retained Reissner's fiber into adulthood could be undertaken. Attractive candidates for such a search would include those who have had some type of paranormal or mystical experience, such as a near-death experience, synchronicity, or precognition. A 2009 poll showed that 49% of Americans had a mystical experience defined as a "moment of sudden religious insight or awakening." Interestingly, in 1992 only 22% reported such experiences.

Once suitable subjects have been developed or identified, various methods could be used to enhance interoceptions of the fiber. Meditation, which quiets external sensory stimulation, could promote such awareness. Indeed mysticism derives from the Greek root *myein*, meaning "to shut the eyes."

However, the mysticism proposed here differs from mysticism as interpreted from conventional psychological perspectives, Eastern philosophies, and recent neuropsychological investigations. Whether mystical experiences are interpreted as regressions to what Freud called the "oceanic feeling" prior to the separation and individuation of the ego, or transcendence according to Buddhist or Hindu philosophies, the dissolution of the ego has been regarded as their hallmark.

Recently, Andrew Newberg, of the Radiology Department at the University of Pennsylvania, and his late colleague of the Psychiatry Department, Dr. Eugene d'Aquili, performed Single Photon Emission Computed Tomography (SPECT) scans of the brains of Buddhist meditators and Franciscan nuns engaged in prayer. When these subjects achieved a "state of pure awareness without the perception of discrete reality, without the sense of the passage of time, without the sense of the extension of space," which the investigators dubbed Absolute Unitary Being (AUB), the scans revealed deafferentiation of the right and left posterior parietal lobes. These experiences suggest nullification of sensory and cognitive functions, *not* supersensory perceptions of transcendent realties. They are like the quieting of the audience and the darkening of the theater before the actual performance begins.

The mysticism proposed here is not dissolution of the ego into an ocean of undifferentiated awareness but its elevation to a uniquely individual infinite "I" who engages in an active dialogue with the Absolute. The neuropsychological basis of this mystical experience is direct consciousness of the subtlest physical activities of Reissner's fiber currently grasped as multidimensional mathematical abstractions and infinities.

Imaging devices capable of measuring Reissner's fiber's activity could provide biofeedback and lead to voluntary control of those activities. Measurement of the fiber's quantum effects could allow the volitional enhancement of quantum coherences. This would be the ultimate goal of the exploration of Reissner's fiber's role in human consciousness; measurement of the fiber's quantum activity and volitional control of it. At the end of our exploration, we might arrive at the place from which it all started 13.82 billion years ago and know it for the first time, discover supernal realities or encounter a physical curiosity unrelated to human consciousness.

First Steps Along the Road

In 2000, in a new opportunity to re-enter the road that had ended for me forty years earlier presented itself. Peretz Lavie, President, Technion-Israel Institute of Technology, introduced me to Dr. Irina Zhdanova, Professor in the Department of Anatomy and Neurobiology, Boston University School of Medicine, whose research on the pineal gland had led to her rare acquaintance with Reissner's fiber. Trying to find a middle ground between pie in the sky speculation and meaningless data collection, we agreed that developing a transgenic zebrafish whose Reissner's fiber would incorporate green fluorescent protein (GFP) would be a suitable first step. First, we tried to incorporate GFP into F-spondin, a protein associated with the fiber. But this hybrid proved to be unstable. Eventually after thousands of hours of DNA splicing, breeding, and analyzing we created a transgenic zebrafish in which in which the expression of GFP is under control of the promoter for F-spondin. This effective visual tool has allowed for detailed neuroanatomical localization of F-spondin, and helps us focus on Reissner's fiber in living animals.

F-spondin is involved with adult neurogenesis, the birth of new neurons in a mature brain and their incorporation into active neuronal circuits involved in cognitive and emotional processes. It also suppresses the production of amyloid protein that is associated with the pathogenesis of Alzheimer's disease. We are using advanced physical and mathematical modeling to investigate kinetics and dynamics of adult neurogenesis, including the cell division cycle, cell migration, and differentiation into functional neurons. We are also exploring the epigenetics factors involved in the expression of F-spondin with the hope of better understanding its typical fetal involution in humans.

While our research holds the promise of developing prophylactics of age-dependent decline in cognitive functions, and treatment strategies for brain traumas or neurodegenerative disorders, I still wanted to follow my quantum mystical dreams. It had been forty years since I had glimpsed Reissner's fiber sliding off my makeshift hook as I prepared to investigate its quantum properties using Dr. Loeser's time-resolved ultra-fast fluorescent microscope. For twenty-five years, as a practicing psychiatrist, I tried to realize my dream of once again traveling along the road I had started as a medical student by writing essays and articles and communicating with scientists. But quantum biology was dismissed as a pipe dream and Reissner's fiber was concealed beneath the Devil's cloak.

Quantum mysticism peaked in the 1950s, and following the deaths of Schrödinger, Pauli, Arthur Eddington, and James Jeans the subject of the relationship between consciousness and quantum theory was largely dismissed by scientists as "quantum woo". However, new technologies that far surpass those of the 1970s have recently created bridges between biology and quantum mechanics. Googling various keywords as a modern day form of logomancy, I was directed to Professor Alexander Sergienko's website. He is a professor in the Department of Electrical and Computer Engineering and Department of Physics at Boston University Photonics Center, working on "Ultra-precise optical measurement in science and technology, Quantum nanoscale sensors and sensor networks, and Quantum bio-photonics."

Intrigued by our photomicrographs of green fluorescent pathways in the retina and the core of the brain, and comparing mainstream physics to "sweeping dust around the corners," Professor Sergienko agreed to help us search for possible quantum effects in Reissner's fiber. The goal of our research is to develop an instrument capable of measuring photon emissions from Reissner's fiber with sufficient resolution and sensitivity to detect possible classical and non-classical signals.

Entering the basement lab through a revolving door, like the one I had walked through to enter Dr. Loeser's lab forty years earlier, I feel as if have been transported into the future. A year after our first discussions, our team developed a prototype. A confocal microscope with customized filters, a customized quartz cuvette to provide additional filtering and nanopositioners and stabilizers is positioned above zebrafish larvae embedded in agar. Photons received by the microscope are transmitted to a novel superconducting single photon detector (SSPD). The active element of the SSPD is a meander-shaped narrow stripe covering the 10x10 micrometer area. The stripe is fabricated from a 4-nanometer thick superconducting Nobium Nitride film that has been spattered on a double-side polished sapphire substrate using the direct electron-beam lithography and reactive ion etching. Signals from the SSPD are analyzed by a time correlated single Photon Counting (TCSP) system with picosecond resolution. Femtosecond pulsed infrared lasers can excite the fiber and perform photon echo-based experiments similar to those recently used to reveal the quantum mechanisms involved in light harvesting during photosynthesis. Using transgenic zebrafish with genetically encoded calcium indicators, we can document neuronal activity associated with quantum behaviors in the fiber. Our zebrafish facility is also equipped for video monitoring and computerized analysis of behaviors.

Drifting back to my adolescent quantum mystical dreams, I imagine twin mirrors reflecting the frontiers of the future and the origin of the past. The lost secrets of the interoceptions of Reissner's fiber engraved in sapphire by the angel Raziel and the photonic signals from the fiber in Casper zebrafish stimulating 4-nanometer thick superconducting Nobium Nitride film that has been spattered on a double-side polished sapphire substrate using the direct electron-beam lithography and reactive ion etching stand poised to unite science and religion. But the presence of a mysterious Being, "who was of all living beings the most interested in the destruction of Superstition," and who "didn't disdain to inspire the pens, words and the consciences of all pedagogues ... at all the scientific meetings," had followed me into that "subterranean dwelling" and wakened me from my dream. But I'm still dreaming.

An optimistic forecast for our experiment would be measurements of quantum coherence beyond the 300 femtoseconds that have been observed in photosynthetic systems. This spark of quantum coherence might ignite the fires of imagination in a few scientists.

Besides looking for quantum coherences that could amplify quantum mechanical interactions with the one-dimensional thread running through the fiber's hollow core and facilitate interactions with classical neural events, we are also developing mathematical models of the fiber. Dimitri Nanopoulos and Nick Mavromatos have developed string theoretic models of microtubules that are applicable to Reissner's fiber. Illuminating the frontiers of the interaction between Reissner's fiber and the one-dimensional string running through its hollow core is "monstrous moonshine." Which derives its name from the inexplicable correspondence between the coefficients of the "monster group," which consists of 808,017,424,794,512,875,886,459,904,961,710,757,005,754,368, 000,000,000 elements formed by rotations in a 196,883-dimensional space, and the coefficients of a complex variety of elliptic function called the j-function. Physicists, including Edward Witten, have bridged the correspondence of "monstrous moonshine" with string theory. While black holes and the initial singularity have received the most attention as testing grounds for exotic applications of string theory, Reissner's fiber could provide an even more exotic laboratory. Perhaps the two-dimensional holographic encoding of the universe could be encoded onto the one-dimensional thread running through the center of Reissner's fiber.

Clues for creating a neurocosmological laboratory organized around the one-dimensional thread running through the hollow core of the fiber could come from recent experimental evidence of a one-dimensional Luttinger fluid[1] within a carbon nanotube. The abstract mathematical models describing one-dimensional quantum systems in condensed matter have been spectacularly confirmed. Stephan Stojkovic's theory that the early universe had one spatial dimension, that could resolve the current incompatibilities between general relativity and quantum mechanics, might also provide clues. Because gravity waves could not have propagated in the proposed one-dimensional early universe, the theory could be tested by gravity wave detectors such as the Laser Interferometer Space Antenna (LISA) scheduled to be launched in the 2030s.

Interpenetrating the labyrinthine paths from possible quantum coherences measurable by biophoton emissions to gravity are the weak and strong nuclear forces. What is the connection between the parity violations of the weak nuclear and biological chirality and cerebral laterality? Do the fractional charges of quarks involve "subquantum" phenomena? How is consciousness related to the Higgs field, dark energy, and dark matter?

The road toward the realization and verification of a unified neurocosmology organized around Reissner's fiber, if there is such a road, is long. Two centuries is a reasonable estimate for completing the journey. Femtosecond infrared pulses reflecting a green fluorescent glow illuminate an unmovable finger obstinately pointing to God.

But those lights might reveal only noise from a waste disposal system, or from a phylogentically ancient morphogenetic structure that involutes in humans before birth. The unmovable finger obstinately pointing beyond quantum mechanics to consciousness, Hindu scriptures, and God might be pointing to empty metaphysics and wishful thinking. Quantum mechanics might be only trivially related to consciousness. The parallels between modern physics and Hindu scriptures might simply reflect the fact that ultimate reality transcends the kaleidoscopic, finite self-referential web of language. The "subtle anatomy" might represent primitive anthropomorphic conceptions of God. God might be an illusion. Divine Providence, an absolute moral order, and eternal life after death are merely the way we wish things to be.

---

[1] A Luttinger fluid is a theoretical model describing electrons in a one-dimensional conductor such as carbon nanotubes.

Reissner's fiber could provide a tangible touchstone for determining if religion is true.

Giving the Devil His Due

The Talmud tells us everything Satan does he does for the sake of heaven. Reissner's fiber as the Devil according to Baudelaire is consistent with Talmudic wisdom.

Owing to God's absolute infinitude, He and the Devil are one.

Ever since the Devil enticed Eve to eat from the forbidden fruit of the Tree of Knowledge, God has exiled us from our paradisiacal union with Him. Humankind has struggled in a world of suffering and death. While Job proclaimed, "Yet from my flesh I shall see God," he beseeched the Lord to explain his unjust suffering. God replied, "Who is this that obscures my plans with words without knowledge? ... Where were you when I laid the earth's foundation? ... What is the way to the abode of light? And where does darkness reside?" The tension between good and evil, between God and the Devil, rests in our ignorance. If we can open the doors of perception to the Infinite, then we can align our will with God.

But if Reissner's fiber is our lost circuit to heaven, why did God make the road to salvation so long and difficult? The answer is that interoceptions of the fiber by the circumneurocelic sensory system and exteroceptions by neuroimaging devices must be perfectly balanced. An imbalance could be catastrophic. Just as God fine-tuned the cosmological constant beyond the hundredth decimal point to create a habitable universe, so too must we perfectly balance our consciousness of the fiber. For now, Reissner's fiber must play its trick of convincing us that it doesn't exist.

Perception of the fiber by the circumneurocelic sensory system alone could lead to a regression to humankind's infancy prior to the commission of the metaphysical original sin and the separation and individuation of the ego. To the extent that an individual's consciousness is dominated by interoceptions of Reissner's fiber, it is submerged in the evolutionary ancient era of programmed reactivity. That era ended with the commission of the metaphysical original sin and the start of the journey along the road of science.

Prophets from Moses to Elijah, Buddha, and Lao-Tse bridged the abyss between our primal origins and our leap toward transcendence. But the era of prophecy has ended. Human creativity and reason have supplanted divine revelation. Prophets are no longer integrable into society.

Exteroception of the fiber by neuroimaging devices alone would decouple our experience of the fiber from interoceptive consciousness of the fiber. Such a decoupling—if the identification of the fiber with the "subtle anatomy" is true—would perpetuate the separation from our cosmogenic source.

According to the latest cosmological models based on inflation and Higgs fields, the universe can be visualized as a "Mexican hat." Our current universe is in a "metastable" state, the lowest energy level corresponding to the dip below the brim of the hat. The universe has been stable for 13.8 billion years because there is insufficient energy to climb over the brim and plunge to a lower level. However, quantum tunneling provides a non-classical mechanism for surmounting an energy barrier. It provides an explanation for the triggering of the inflationary expansion of the Higgs vacuum 13.8 billion years ago. The probability of tunneling through the Higgs vacuum is very small. But volitional control of quantum coherences in Reissner's fiber might make such tunneling possible. The Biblical promise of a new heaven and earth could be realized in a universe over the brim of the "Mexican hat." The Devil's mission would be to prevent the vacuum's premature reconfiguration by a short circuit between Reissner's fiber and the vacuum. Harnessing the energy of the physical vacuum, (*calculated* to be 10^{113} ergs/cm^3), could trigger explosions that would make the world's nuclear arsenal look like a flaming arrow shot by a medieval archer.

Reissner's fiber has thwarted its identification with the "subtle anatomy" because the Devil, in its role as the destroyer of superstitions, has successfully, thus far, convinced scientists that the "subtle anatomy" is a superstition rather than a factual description of interoceptions. This has been my experience with scientists, with rare exceptions, since Eccles expressed his alarm.

Not only has Reissner's fiber thwarted its identification with the "subtle anatomy" by relegating ancient interoceptions to the realm of fantastical superstitions, but it has also thwarted the identification by hiding in plain sight. Recently, adding to the strange tales of Sargent, Enami, Bonghan, Rele, and Bernard, Reissner's fiber flamboyantly flaunted its trick of convincing us that it does not exist. In September 15, 2009, Dan Brown, after years of research, published *The Lost Symbol*. It had a first printing of 6.5 million. On its first day the book sold one million in hardcover and e-book versions, making it the fastest selling adult novel in history. There are more than 30 million copies in print worldwide.

Near the novel's conclusion, Katherine, a character who conducts experiments in noetic science, tells the hero, Robert Langdon:

> Perhaps you've heard ... abut the brain of yogis while they mediate? The human brain, in advanced states of focus, will physically create a waxlike substance from the pineal gland. This brain secretion is unlike anything else in the body. It has an incredible healing effect, can literally regenerate cells, and may be one of the reasons yogis live so long. This is real science, Robert. This substance has inconceivable properties and can be created only by a mind highly tuned to a deeply focused state.

This "waxlike substance" corresponds almost exactly to Reissner fiber which is secreted from the pineal-subcommissural organ. Its effects on regenerating the severed tails of tadpoles and zebrafish are well documented. It "can literally regenerate cells." It is intimately connected with the biological clock and may be one of the reasons yogis live so long. A mind highly tuned the fiber's quantum mechanical effects by the inner directed sensory system surrounding would endow this substance with "inconceivable properties."

On June 7, 2014, I met Dan Brown at a reception at the Mark Twain House in Hartford, Connecticut. He was amazed and excited to hear that the waxy substance secreted by the pineal is real. Neither he nor any of his millions of readers had previously pointed out the correspondence to Reissner's fiber. Critics and bloggers had mocked his "pseudoscientific pretensions."

The connection between Reissner's fiber and speculations about quantum theories, including string theories and other attempts to include gravity, has been thwarted by the limits of our understanding of the quantum mechanics of composite systems. Only small progress has been made since 1922 when Einstein observed that we are still "far away from being able to convert these vague ideas into a theory." Even if an adequate theory for modeling Reissner's fiber were available, we're still far away from developing technologies that could confirm the predictions of such a theory.

Shortly after he had unified various versions of string theory, which postulates one-dimensional strings and multidimensional objects of infinite extension called "branes," into a theory called "M-theory," I called Edward Witten at his office at the Institute for Advanced Study in Princeton. Held in awe in by his colleagues for his mathematical prowess, Witten had cryptically said that the "M" stands from "magical, mysterious, or murky."

While Witten and his fellow string theorists dominate theoretical physics, many physicists have become critical of the theory. Some physicists insist the "M" stands for "medieval theology." String theorists, they say, are like theologians counting angels on the head of a pin. The theory has yet to make any empirically testable predictions.

I suggested to Dr. Witten that Reissner's fiber could provide testable predictions of M-theory. The brain's enormous computational powers and precise, coordinated control of its 100 billion electrical components could be harnessed to promote quantum coherences in the fiber. The ventricular cavities of the brain could be analogous to the quantum electrodynamic cavities that use feedback and control to produce such coherences. Might the strings comprising Reissner's fiber thereby condense and thereby greatly amplify their effects? Would it be possible to develop a mathematical model of such macroscopic condensation of strings? Witten, who would go on develop correspondences between "monstrous moonshine" and 194 varieties of black holes, listened intently. After a lengthy pause and a deep sigh, he told me my ideas about Reissner's fiber were "too exotic" for him. While the recent discovery of quantum coherences in biological systems has lowered the barriers of skepticism, the gap between branes and brains remains unbridged.

Einstein once observed, "It is easier to denature plutonium than to denature the evil spirit of man." He also believed that "knowledge of what *is* does not open the door directly to what *should be*." His road of science stopped at the threshold of morality.

But Einstein stood before a door that might directly lead from what *is* to what *should be*. Spinoza's vision of attaining a level of knowledge beyond reason, knowing the body under a form of eternity, achieving blessedness, whereby "the love of God towards men and the mind's intellectual love towards God are one and the same," could be fulfilled by synthesizing the old elements of the "subtle anatomy" with the new scientific understandings of Reissner's fiber. This might hold the key to denaturing the evil sprit of man. Einstein stood before the door leading to the path from his scientific paradise to a new religious paradise informed by its ancient roots and illuminated by science. It was a road not traveled.

Physics has peered into the abyss of "the abode of light" and has seen esoteric abstractions suspended in the ether. Reissner's fiber could give substance to that ethereal trail across the abyss and serve as a tightrope.

According to the Kabbalah, the clock recording the time to the end of the final 7,000-year long cycle started to tick on September 7, 3761 BC. According to relativity, the end of our final 7,000-year long cycle is here now, embraced by eternity. Neural activity generates the illusory milliseconds-wide window into eternity. By regenerating the fiber and consciously controlling its activity at the limits of objectivity, we might complete its 500 million year evolutionary journey, enter the Western gate of paradise, and unite the end of the future with the beginning of the past.

Believing in things we don't understand has led to suffering since the commission of the Biblical original sin. By destroying superstition, the Devil keeps us on the road to understanding grounded in reason and empirical facts. Under the watchful eyes of God and the Devil, scientists will no doubt make new clearings along the road of science. But that road has reached a number of impasses. Basic intuitions about form and function tell us that the meter-long Reissner's fiber, surrounded by naked nerve endings and sensory receptors, could create a new circuit in the brain and thereby, for us, create a new reality. Whether that new reality transcends the limits of science is a testable hypothesis.

Bibliography

Agduhr, E. (1922) Uber ein zentrales Sinnesorgan (?) bei den Vertebraten, *Zischr. Anat. Entwickelungesch,* **66**, pp. 223–230.

Avalon, A. (Woodroff, Sir John) (2012) *The Serpent Power,* New Delhi: New Age Books.

Bell, J.S., quoted in: Rosenblum, B., Kuttner, F. (2006) *Quantum Enigma: Physics Encounters Consciousness,* New York: Oxford University Press.

Bernard, T. (1940) *Heaven Lies Within Us,* New York: Rider and Company.

Bohr, N. quoted in: French, A. (1985) *Niels Bohr: A Centenary Volume,* Cambridge, MA: Oxford University Press.

Capra, F. (1975) *The Tao of Physics,* Boston, MA: Shambhala.

Darwin. C. (1881) *The Formation of Vegetable Mould through the Action of Worms, with Observations on their Habits,* London: John Murray.

DeJean, J. (1991) *Tender Geographies: Women and the Origins of the Novel in France,* New York: Columbia University Press.

Dendy, A. (1909) The function of Reissner's fiber and the ependymal groove, *Nature,* **82**.

De Vernejoul, P., et al. (1985) Study of acupuncture meridians using radioactive tracers, *Bulletin de L'Academie Nationale de Medicine,* **169** (7), pp. 1071–1075. (References to Bong Han, Kim J. (1963) *Democratic People's Republic of Korea Academy of Sciences* No. 5; 1965. *Proceedings Academy Kungrak DPRK,* No. 2, Pongyang, Korea: Medical Sciences Press.)

Edinger, L. (1908) Vorlesungen uber den Bau der nervosen Centralorgane des Menschen und der Tiere, *Vergl. Anat. des Gehirnes,* Bd 2, 7, Aufl. Leipzig.

Einstein, A. (1953) *Ideas and Opinions,* New York: Crown Publishers.

Einstein, A. quoted in: Bricmont, J. (2105) *Making Sense of Quantum Mechanics,* Switzerland: Springer International Publishing.

Einstein, A. quoted in: Stachel, J. (2002) *Einstein 'B' to 'Z',* Basel: Verlag.

Enami, M. (1954) Preoptico-subcommissural neurosecretory system in the eel, *Endocrinol. Japon.,* **2** (1), pp. 33–45.

Erbl-Roth, G. (1951) Uberden Reissnerchen Fadender Wirbeltiere, *Zeitscheiff Fur Mickr. Anat. Forsh.*, **57**, pp. 180–195.

Fisher, M. (2015) *Quantum Cognition: The possibility of processing with nuclear spins in the brain*, arXiv: 1508.05929.

Frohlich, H. (1968) Long range coherence and energy storage in biological systems, *Journal of Quantum Chemistry*, **2**, pp. 64–649.

Gadow, H. (1891) *Vogel, Bronn's Klassen und Ordnungen des Thierreichs*, Bd. 8, Abth. 4.

Gödel, K. quoted in: Rucker, R. (2004) *Infinity and the Mind*, Basel: Birkhauser.

Gomez, B., Benito-Aaranz, E. & Rodriguez, M. (1961) The subcommissural organ in the grown-up man, *Acta. Anat.*, **44**, pp. 98–103.

Gordon, D. (2010) *Ant Encounters: Interaction Networks and Colony Behavior*, (Primers in Complex Systems), Princeton, NJ: Princeton University Press.

Greenstein, G. (1988) *The Symbiotic Universe: Life and Mind in the Cosmos*, New York: William Morrow & Co.

Hackett, P. (2012) *Theos Bernard, The White Lama*, New York: Columbia University Press.

Harnard, S. (2008) *What it Feels Like to Hear Voices: Fond Memories of Julian Jaynes*, arXiv: 0808.3563.

Heisenberg, W. quoted in: Herbert, N. (1985) *Quantum Reality: Beyond the New Physics*, Garden City, NY: Anchor Press/Doubleday.

Hess, J. (1973) Studies concerning the function of the complex subcommissural organ-liquor fibre: The binding of the liquor fibre to pyrocatechin derivatives and its functional aspects, *Brain Research*, **58**, pp. 303–312.

Hess, J. & Sterba, G. (1972) Die Bindungsfahigkeit des Reissnerschen Fadens fur Adrenalin und Noradrenalin in vivo, *Acta. Biol. Med. Germ.*, **28**, pp. 849–851.

Horsley, V. (1908) Note on the existence of Reissner's fiber in higher vertebrates, *Brain*, **31** (1), pp. 147–159.

Jastrow, R. (1978) *God and the Astronomers*, New York: W.W. Norton & Co.

Jaynes, J. (1976) *The Origin of Consciousness in the Breakdown of the Bicameral Mind*, Boston, MA: Houghton Mifflin.

Jaynes, J.C. (2015) *Magic Wells: Sermons*, Oxford: Andesite Press.

Jordan, H. (1919) Concerning Reissner's fiber in teleosts, *Journal of Comparative Neurology*, **122**, pp. 216–227.

Kalberlah, T. (1900) Uber das Ruckenmark der Plagiostomen Ein Beitrag sur vergleichenden Anatomies des Centralnervansystems, *Zeitschr. f. ges. Naturwiss*, **73**.

Kaufmann, S. (2012) Answering Descartes: Beyond Turing, in Cooper, D. & Hodges, A. (eds.) *The Once and Future Turing: Computing the World*, Cambridge: Cambridge University Press.

Keene, M.L.F. & Hewer, E.E. (1935) The subcommissural organ and the mesocoelic recess in the human brain, together with a note on Reissner's fibre, *Journal of Anatomy (London)*, **69**, pp. 501–507.

Kohno, K. (1969) Electron microscope study of Reissner's fiber, *Z. Zellforsch*, **94**, pp. 565–573.

Krishna, G. (1970) *Kundalini: The Evolutionary Energy in Man*, Boston, MA: Shambhala Books.

Leatherland, J. & Dodd, J. (1968) Studies on the structure, ultrastructure and function of the subcommissural organ-Reissner's fibre complex of the European eel Anguilla Anguilla L., *Zeitschrift für Zellforschung und Mikroskopische Anatomie*, **89** (4), pp. 553–549.

Lee, B.C., Kim, S. & Soh, K.S. (2008) Novel anatomical structure in the brain and spinal cord of rabbit that may belong the Bonghan system of potential acupuncture meridians, *Journal of Acupuncture Meridian Studies*, **1**, pp. 29–35.

Leggett, A. quoted in: Goswami, A. (1993) *The Self-Aware Universe*, New York: Tarcher.

Marin, J.M. (2009) Mysticism in quantum mechanics: The forgotten controversy, *European Journal of Physics*, **30**, pp. 807–822.

Matthiae, P. (1977) *Ebla; An Empire Rediscovered*, London: Hodder & Stoughton.

Mavromatos, N. & Nanopouluas, D. (1997) *Microtubules: The neuronic system of the neurons?*, arXiv:quant-ph/9702003.

Marx, K. (1998) *The German Ideology. Literary Theory: An Anthology*, Oxford: Blackwell.

Motavkin, P. & Bakhtinov, A. (1990) Intraspinal organ in man, *Arkhiv Anatomii, Gistologii I Embriologii*, **99** (10), pp. 5–19.

Motoyama, H. (2001) *Theories of the Chakras: Bridge to Higher Consciousness*, Madras, India: Quest Books.

Nanopoulos, D. (1995) *Theory of Brain Function, Quantum Mechanics and Superstrings*, arXiv: hep-ph/9505374.

Newberg, A. (2010) *Principles of Neurotheology*, London: Routledge.

Nicholls, G. (1909) The function of Reissner's fiber and the ependymal groove, *Nature*, **82**.

Nicholls, G. (1917) Some experiments on the nature and function of Reissner's fiber, *Journal of Comparative Neurology*, **27** (2), pp. 119–199.

Penrose, R. & Hameroff, S. (2011) Consciousness in the universe: Neuroscience, quantum space-time geometry and Orch OR theory, *Jounral of Cosmology*, **14**.

Perival, I. cited in Einstein's Unknown Insight and the Problem of Quantizing Chaos (2005) Stone, A.D., *Physics Today*.

Pettinato, G. (1991) *Ebla: A New Look at History*, Baltimore, MD: Johns Hopkins University Press.

Ponce, C. (1978.) *Kabbalah*, Wheaton, IL: The Theosophical Publishing House.

Poulin, M. (2013) https://melissareeserpoulin.com/2013/08/31/like-a-tinsmiths-scoop/.

Quine, W. (1964) *Word and Object*, Cambridge, MA: MIT Press.

Rakic, P. (1965) Mesocoelic recess in the human brain, *Neurology*, **15**, pp. 708–715.

Rakic, P. & Sidman, R. (1968) Subcommissural organ and adjacent ependyma: Autoradiographic study of their origin in the mouse brain, *The American Journal of Anatomy*, **122**, pp. 317–336.

Reissner, E. (1860) Beitrage zur Kenntiss vom Bau des Ruskenmarks von Petromyzon fluvatis, *Arch. Anat. Physiol*, pp. 445–488.

Rele, V.G. (2007) *Mysterious Kundalini*, Delhi: Bhrativa Kala Prakashan.

Rohon, J.V. (1870) Das Centralorgan des Nervensystems der Selachier, *Deks Acad. Wiss. Wien Math. Naturw*, Bd. 38.

Sanders, A. (1878) Contribution to the anatomy of the central nervous system in vertebrate animals, *Philosophical Transactions Royal Society London*, **189**.

Sanders, A. (1894) Researches in the nervous system of *Myxine glutinosa*, *Philsophical Transactions Royal Society London*.

Sargent, P.E. (1900) Reissner's fiber in the canalis centralis of vertebrates, *Anat. Anz, Bd*, 17.

Sargent, P.E. (1905) The optic reflex apparatus of vertebrates for short-circuit transmission of motor reflexes through Reissner's fiber: Its morphology, ontogeny, phylogeny and function. Part I. The fish-like vertebrates, *Bulletin of the Museum of Comparative Zoology at Harvard University*, **45**, pp. 1–256.

Schrödinger, E. (1969) *What is Life? and Mind and Matter*, Cambridge: Cambridge University Press.

Snell, B. (1953) *The Discovery of the Mind: The Greek Origins of European Thought*, Cambridge, MA: Harvard University Press.

Soh, K.S. (2004) Bonghan duct and acupuncture meridian as optical channel of biophotons, *Journal of the Korean Physical Society*, **45** (5), pp. 1196–1198.

Soh, K.S. (2009) Bonghan circulatory system as an extension of acupuncture meridians, *J Acupunct Meridian Stud,* **2** (2), pp. 93–106.

Stapp, H., Schwartz, J.M & Beauregard, M. (2005) Quantum theory in neuroscience and psychology: A neurophysical model of mind-brain interaction, *Philosophical Transactions of the Royal Society of London,* Series B, **360** (1458), pp. 1309–1327.

Stieda, L. (1868) Studien uber des centrale Neuroensystem des Wirbelthiere, *Zeits. f. wiss. Zool.,* **19**.

Stojkovic, S. (2013) *Vanishing dimensions: theory and phenomenology,* ArXiv: 1304.6444.

Streeter, G.L. (1902) The structure of the spinal cord of the ostrich, *American Journal of Anatomy,* **3**.

Studnicka, F.K. (1899) Der Reissner'schen Faden aus Centralcanal des Ruckenmarks und sein Verhalken in dem Ventriculus (sinus) terminalis, *Sitzb. k. bahm Ges. Wiss. math. Nat.,* Kl. Prag.

Susskind, L. (2005) *The Cosmic Landscape: String Theory and the Illusion of Intelligent Design,* Boston, MA: Little, Brown &Co.

Swedenborg, E. (1976) *The Fibre,* Bryn Athyn, PA: Swedenborg Scientific Association.

Tipler, F. (2007) *The Physics of Christianity,* New York: Doubleday.

Tolstoy, L. (1899) *What is Art?,* New York: Thomas Y. Crowell & Co.

Vitay, G., Kaufmann, S. & Niiranaen, S. (2012) *Quantum biology on the edge of quantum chaos,* arXiv: 1202.6433.

Viault, F. (1876) Recherches histologiques sur la Strucuture des Centres nerveux des Plagiostomes, *Arch. Zool. exper. gen,* Tom. 5.

Vilkov, G. (1980) Detection of neurotropic properties of the serum in schizophrenics, translated from *Zhurnal Nevropatologii i Psikiatriii imeni S. S. Koraakova,* **80** (1), pp. 67–70.

Vishnu-devananda, S. (1960) *The Complete Illustrated Book of Yoga,* New York: Three Rivers Press.

Vivekananda, S. (1947) *Complete Works of Swami Vivekananda volume 1,* Advaita Ashrara.

Wile, L. (1994) Near-death experiences: A speculative neural model, *Journal of Near-Death Studies,* **12** (3), pp. 133–142.

Wile, L. (2016) Reissner's fibre: A forgotten pathway for exploring consciousness, *Journal of Consciousness Studies,* **23** (3–4), pp. 191–211.

Witten, E., *Three-Dimensional Gravity Revisited,* arXiv: 0706.3359 [hep-th].

Woolam, D.H.M. (1982) The circumventricular organs of the brain: Their possible role as sites for future neurosurgery, *Annals of the Royal College of Surgeons of England,* **64**, pp. 310–317.

Woolam, D.H.M. & Collins, P. (1980) Reissner's fibre in the rat: A scanning and transmission electron microscope study, *Journal Anatomy London,* **131**, pp. 135–143.

Yogananda, P. (1995) *Autobiography of a Yogi,* Los Angeles, CA: Self Realization Fellowship.

Yogananda, P. (1997) *God Talks With Arjuna: The Bhagavad Gita,* Los Angeles, CA: Self Realization Fellowship.

Index

Abhedananda, 142
Abraham (Genesis), 162, 165
absolute knowledge, 111, 117, 118
Abulafia, Abraham, 105
acupuncture, 3, 73, 144–148
Adam and Eve (Genesis), 26, 126, 165
Adam Kadmon, 106, 111, 115, 122, 130–131
Adiyoga, 122
Agduhr, Eric, 87, 88–89
Ahab, King of Israel, 29, 168
ajna chakra (yoga), 73
Akiva ben Yosef, 129
Alexander, Samuel, 6
Amos (prophet), 25–26, 30, 159–160, 161
analog "I", 5, 16–17, 21–22, 31, 45
Angel of Conception (Lailah), 122
anterior commissure, 18–19, 39
Anthropic Principle, 123–124
archeological evidence, 20, 22, 162–163, 164–165
Aristotle, 15, 47
Ark of the Covenant, 126–127
arum (Hebrew word), 26
asanas (yoga), 138–139
assimilation (Piaget), 55–56
associationism, 37
Assyrian archeology, 22
atom, Bohr model, 58
auditory hallucinations. *see also* bicameral mind
  broadcast to other people, 42
  as effect of language comprehension, 19
  in Old Testament, 165–169, 171
  in origin of Jaynes's theory, 36, 37, 39
  as origin of Jaynesian consciousness, 5, 55–57, 171
  possession (spiritual), 31
  schizophrenia, 5, 18, 29, 32–34, 49, 170–171
  and social order, 20–22, 53–54
Axelrod, Julius, 153
Ayers, Howard, 82

Baal Shem Tov, 131
Bakhtinov, A.P., 85
Basange, Jacques, 105
Baudelaire, Charles, 76
Bauer, Edmond, 66
Beck, Friedrich, 70
Beckenstein, Jacob, 69
behaviorism, 9–10, 12–13, 37–39, 42, 43
Bell, J.S., 61, 62, 67–68
Bell's Inequality, 61
Beltran, Miquel, 106
Bernard, Theos, 140–143, 156
Bernstein, Julius, 84
Besso, Michael, 60, 61, 91, 93
Bible
  bicameral mind in, 25–30, 159–169
  Einstein on, 102
  Freud's gift from father, 113, 117
  Gospels, 128
  Newton on, 108–109
  Old Testament, 25–30, 110, 128–129, 159–169
  Spinoza on, 109–110
  Swedenborg on, 77–78
  Torah, 110, 126–127
bicameral mind. *see also* auditory hallucinations

breakdown, 21–30, 159, 161–162, 165–169
  of civilizations, 53–54
  "general paradigm", 31
  Greek gods, 18, 49–51
  Hebrew god(s), 24–30, 163–167
  Jaynes's development of theory, 38–40
  neural substrate, 18–19
  vestiges in modern world, 31–33
Big Bang, 99. *see also* initial singularity
Blavatsky, Madame, 152
Bloch, Chayim, 114–115
Bloch, Joseph, 115
body regulation, 128–129, 136–137, 176
Bohm, David, 69
Bohr, Niels, 58, 60, 63–65
Bonghan system, 145, 146, 147–148
Born, Max, 60, 61
Bose, Satyendra Nath, 119
Bose-Einstein condensations, 119
Brahma nadi (yoga), 134, 135, 154
Brahma-randhra (yoga), 134, 136, 143–144
brain. *see also* Reissner's fiber; subcommissural organ (SCO)
  basis for bicameral mind, 18–19, 54
  body regulation, 128–129, 136–137
  circumneurocelic sensory system, 88–93
  embryonic development, 150–154
  location of consciousness, 47–48, 57–58
  structure, 151–154
Breuer, Josef, 112
Broca's area, 47
Broch, Hermann, 109
Broglie, Louis de, 60
Brown, Dan, 182–183
Brucke, Ernst, 78
Buchner, Ludwig, 103

Cantor, Georg, 99–100
Cantor's infinites, 99–100

Capra, Fritjof, 72
Casimir effect, 93
central canal, 143–144, 149–150
cerebrospinal fluid (CSF)
  CSF-contacting neurons, 88–89, 92
  early studies, 80
  effect of yoga, 139, 175
  history, 150–151
  in hydrocephalus, 86–87
  as "liquor cerebrospinalis", 155
chakras (yoga), 3, 73–74, 133–134, 136
Chasidism, 111, 113–114, 131
Chinese medicine, 3, 73–74, 122, 144–148, 171
Chittra nadi (yoga), 134, 135, 141, 142–144, 154
Chomsky, Noam, 98
Choose Life (Gutkind), 109
circumneurocelic sensory system, 88–93, 181
circumventricular organs, 89
civilization clashes and bicameral breakdown, 21–22, 24
Cohanim, 163
Cohen, I.B., 109
collective cognitive imperative, 31, 42
concepts, 12, 37, 42
conciliation, 17
conditioned learning, 12–13, 37–38, 43. *see also* behaviorism
consciousness
  and behaviorism, 37–39
  and body regulation, 136–137
  eternal nature of, 2–3, 172–174
  evolution, 1–2, 170, 173
  experiments, 13, 37–38, 43
  holographic model, 69–70
  location, 46–48, 57–58, 63, 71–72, 74, 83. *see also* brain
  perception of quantum world, 72–73, 90–94
  quantum mechanical basis of, 57–60, 63–66, 68–72, 118–120, 129–130
  religious texts as sources on, 1, 3
  theories of, 6–15

unconscious processes behind, 43
consciousness, Jaynesian
  defined, 1–2
  definition of "concepts", 42–43
  features, 16–17
  free will, 46
  location, 15, 46–48
  as metaphor, 5–6, 15–16
  origin, 21–30, 54–57, 160–161
  perception, 41–42
consciousness of consciousness, 2, 11, 41–42, 43–46, 52, 172. *see also* strange loops
continuity hypothesis (Darwin), 7–8
Copenhagen Interpretation, 58–59, 67
Cordovero, Moses ben Jacob, 105–106, 130
Correspondence Principle, 118
cosmic landscapes theory, 124
cosmological constant, 99, 123
CSF-contacting neurons, 88–89, 92

Dan, Joseph, 131
Darwin, Charles, 7–8, 125
Darwinism, 33, 124–125
David, King of Israel, 28–29
Dawkins, Richard, 1
The Death of Virgil (Broch), 109
deceit as sign of consciousness, 21, 26, 49, 160, 162
DeJean, Joan, 49
Descartes, René, 10, 152
Deshbandhu, 136–137
determinism, universal, 101
Devananda, Vishnu, 154
Devil's Trick, 76, 155, 181–182
diencephalon, 150, 151–152
digital infinity of language, 2–3, 98, 173
Dirac, Paul, 120
The Discovery of Mind (Snell), 51–53
divination, 22, 28
Dodd, J., 84
Dowling, Levi H., 142

Ebla tablets, 164–165
Eccles, Sir John, 70, 156–157
Ecclesiastes, 25–26, 30, 160–161
The Economy of the Animal Kingdom (Swedenborg), 77
Edinger, Ludwig, 82
Egypt, 56, 150
Ein-Sof (Kabbalah), 106, 173, 174
Einstein, Albert
  cosmological constant, 99
  epistemology, 95–98
  flash of insight, 43
  and Freud, 111, 114, 116, 117
  on God and religion, 98–99, 100–104, 106–111, 120–121, 184
  on mathematics, 100
  on philosophy, 172
  on quantum mechanics, 59–63, 64–65, 90–91, 118–119
  on relativity, 96–97, 99
Einstein-Podolsky-Rosen paradox, 61–62
Elijah (prophet), 30, 128
Elijah ben Shlomo Zalman, 131
Elohim (Hebrew God), 26, 30, 105, 163, 164, 167
embryonic development of brain, 150–154
emergentism, 1–2, 9, 55, 56
Enami, Masashi, 84–85
entanglement, 61–62
epithalamus, 152
Ethics (Spinoza), 105
eureka moments (flashes of insight), 14
experience, consciousness as a copy of, 11–12

The Fall (Genesis), 26, 161–162, 173, 181
Feynman, Richard, 67
Fisher, Henry, 69
flashlight analogy (Jaynes), 11, 44
Fliess, Wilhelm, 111–112
Fonesaca, Isaac Aboab da, 105
Force and Matter (Buchner), 103
Francke, A.H., 142
free will, 46, 49–50, 70, 121, 172, 174
Freud, Jakob, 111–112
Freud, Sigmund, 78–79, 111–117

Friedman, Alexander, 99
Fröhlich, Herbert, 68
F-spondin, 85–86, 179
Future of an Illusion (Freud), 117

Gabor, Dennis, 69–70
Galen (Greek physician), 151
Galvani, Luigi, 84
Gardner, James, 138–139
Gauss, Carl Friedrich, 14
gematria (Kabbalah), 105
general bicameral paradigm, 31
Genesis, 25–28, 126–128, 161–163, 165–166
The German Ideology (Marx), 55
glossolalia, 32
God
    Anthropic Principle's implications, 123–124
    and bicameral breakdown, 26–30
    Cantor's infinities, 99–100
    as Designer, 157
    in Ecclesiastes, 161
    Einstein on, 98, 101–104, 107–111, 120, 174, 184
    Elohim, 26, 30, 105, 163, 164, 167
    and free will, 46
    as "I", 46
    Luria on, 130
    perception of, 73–75
    response to Job, 181
    science as search for, 33, 36–40, 95, 174, 180
    Shekinah, 115
    Spinoza on, 104–107, 184
    Yahweh, 26, 163–165, 166, 167
Gödel, Kurt, 44–45, 68
gods, bicameral. *see* bicameral mind
gods, Greek, 17–18, 23–24, 48–51, 56, 161–162
gods, Vedic, 139–140
Gomez, Bosque, 88
Gordon, Deborah, 53–54
Gospels, 128, 129
Governing Vessel, 144, 146, 148
The Grammar of Science (Pearson), 59
gravity, 68–69, 180

Great Human Irony, 33, 40, 94
Greenstein, Georg, 124
gunpowder analogy (Einstein), 90–91
Gutkind, Eric B., 109

Hackett, Paul, 141, 142
Hadamard, Jacques, 96
Haines, Duane, 76, 155
hallucinations, auditory. *see* auditory hallucinations
hallucinations, visual, 27, 166
Hameroff, Stuart, 68
Hammurabi, 21
Hananiah (Book of Jeremiah), 168–169
Harnad, Stevan, 37
Heaney, Seamus, 56
Hebrew people, 24–30, 162–164
Heisenberg, Werner, 58–59, 60, 63, 90
Helmholtz, Hermann von, 14, 33
helpless spectator theory, 8, 46
Herodotus, 50, 56
Herrera, Abraham, 105, 108
Hesiod, 49, 50
Hess, Johann, 155
Hezekiah, King of Judah, 160–161
Hilbert, David, 100
Hinduism, 30, 72–74. *see also kundalini*
Hippocrates, 151
Hofstadter, Douglas, 37
Holographic Principle, 69–70
Homer, 48–52. *see also Iliad; Odyssey*
Hooker, Joseph, 125
Horowitz, Isaac, 127
Horsley, Sir Victor, 82
Hubble, Edwin, 99
Huxley, Thomas, 8, 124
hydrocephalus, 86–87
hypnosis, 32
hypothalamus, 152

"I", philosophical, 45–46. *see also* analog "I"
Idel, Moshe, 131
idols, 20–21, 29, 31
Iliad, 17–18, 23–24, 48–51, 56
Imhotep (Egyptian chancellor), 150

infinities, 98–100
initial singularity, 2, 99, 123, 125, 172, 173
insect colonies, 53–54
insight, flashes of, 14, 43
intuitive knowledge, 104
Is Poetry a Secretion? (Sargent), 81
Isaac of Akko, 123

Jackson, Frank, 89
Jacob (Genesis), 162
Jahn, Robert, 71
Jahoshaphat, King of Judah, 29, 168
James, William, 8
Jastrow, Robert, 123
Jaynes, Julian
    behaviorism, 9–10, 37–39
    develops bicameral theory, 38–40
    father's legacy, 35, 36, 39
    on metaphor, 94–95
    on poetry, 5–6, 23
    on schizophrenia, 170–171
    on science, 94–95, 120, 174
    on theories of consciousness, 6–15
Jaynes, Julian Clifford, 35, 36, 39, 171
Jaynesian consciousness. *see* consciousness, Jaynesian
Jeremiah (prophet), 28, 30, 168–169
Jesus of Nazareth, 106, 128, 129, 141
Joan of Arc, 50
Job (Bible), 181
Jones, Ernst, 78
Jordan, Hovey, 84
Josiah, King of Judah, 25, 167
Jung, Carl, 114

Kabbalah
    cycles of time, 184
    Einstein's inquiries into, 107
    in Freud's life, 111–115
    history, 129–131
    and Reissner's fiber, 122–123, 130–132
    Spinoza on, 104–107
    subtle anatomy in, 3, 73–74
    on the Torah, 126–127
    Zohar, 110, 115, 129–131
Kant, Immanuel, 45
Kapitza, Pyotr, 119
Kaufmann, Stuart, 71
Keene, Lucas, 87
Kent, Adrian, 71
Keynes, John Maynard, 108
khabiru (Assyrian word), 24–25, 28, 162–163
Kim Bong Han, 145–148
Kim Hyun Sik, 146
Kim Il Sung, 145, 146
King, Martin Luther, Jr., 160
knowledge, absolute, 111, 117, 118
knowledge, intuitive, 104
Kölliker, Rudolf Albert von, 83
Kolmer, William, 80, 88–89
Kolmer-Agduhr cells, 89
Krishna, Gopi, 143
kundalini. *see also* yoga
    defined, 73–74
    and Freud, 114, 117
    physical basis, 74, 132–144, 153–158
    possible experiments, 171
Kurkh Monoliths, 163
Kutschin, Karl, 76, 79
Kyungrak Research Institute, 145–146

Lailah, Angel of Conception, 122
Language
    in the bicameral mind, 17–19, 21
    and development of consciousness, 23–24, 55
    digital infinity, 2–3, 98, 173
    evolution of, 2–3, 19, 23–24, 48–49, 98
    as limit on consciousness, 45
    metaphor as ground of, 15–16
Laser Interferometer Space Antenna, 180
Lavie, Peretz, 179
Leadbeater, C.W., 152
learning, relationship of consciousness to, 7–8, 12–13
Leatherland, J., 84
Lee Byung Cheon, 147

Legait, Etienne-Jules, 88
Leggett, Sir Anthony, 67
Lerner, Aaron, 152–153
Lipkin, Daniel, 60–61
liquor cerebrospinalis, 155
lithium isotopes, 69
Locke, John, 37
Loeser, Charles, 85, 148–158
London, Fritz, 66, 119
The Lost Symbol (Brown), 182–183
LSD, 15, 89, 153
Luria, Isaac, 115, 130
Luttinger fluid, 180

Ma'aseh Merkavah, 128
Mad or Muddled (Sargent), 81
Manifesto (1912), 111, 114, 117
Marbe, Karl, 13, 43
Marin, Juan Miguel, 66
Marx, Karl, 33, 55
Matthaie, Paolo, 164
Mavromatos, Nick, 179
meditation, 176, 183
melatonin, 153
Mermin, David, 67
Merneptah Stele, 162
Mesha Stele, 162–163
metaphiers and metaphrands, 6, 15–16, 38, 57
metaphor
  created by consciousness, 56–57
  creator of consciousness, 5–6, 15–16
  in Ecclesiastes, 26
  in Kabbalah, 130–131
  in scientific concepts, 94–95
metaphor "me", 16–17
metaphysical imposition theory, 8, 9, 126
metaphysical original sin, 97–98, 100, 173
Micaiah (prophet), 168
"monstrous moonshine", 179
Mooladra chakra (yoga), 133–134, 136, 153
Moses, 27–28, 126, 127, 128, 165–166
Moses and Monotheism (Freud), 115
Moses de Leon, 129–130

Moszkowski, Alexander, 102
Motavkin, P.A., 85
Motoyama, Hiroshi, 143, 144
M-theory, 183–184
mudras (yoga), 138–139
Muller, Max, 12
multiverse (cosmic landscapes), 124
Muses, Greek, 32
mysticism. *see also* Kabbalah; *kundalini*; yoga
  Freud on, 116
  meditation, 176
  origin, 173
  and quantum mechanics, 64–67, 72–75, 178
  and Reissner's fiber, 87, 90
  and relativity, 111
  as search for direct consciousness, 3

nabiim (Hebrew word), 27, 28, 29–30
nadis (yoga), 3, 73–74, 133–140, 154
Nagel, Thomas, 89
NaNasi, Yehuda, 110
Nanopoulos, Dimitri, 179
narratization, 17
near-death experiences, 47–48, 87, 175–176
Nehunya ben ha-Kanah, 123
Neo-Platonism, 31
Neorealism, 6–7
neural Bonghan duct, 146
neurocele, 2, 85–86, 88, 89, 150, 151, 153
neurocosmology proposition, 3–4, 172
New Immoralities (Sargent), 81
Newberg, Andrew, 176
Newton, Isaac, 107–109, 123–124
Nicholls, George, 83, 135
1912 Manifesto, 111, 114, 117
North Korea, 145–147
Notovitch, Nicholas, 142

Obadiah (prophet), 29–30
Odyssey, 24, 51, 56, 161–162
Ohr-Ein-Sof (Kabbalah), 130

Old Testament, 25–30, 110, 128–129, 159–169
Olry, Regis, 76, 155
On the Origin of Species (Darwin), 125
Onnes, Heike Kamerlingh, 118, 119
oracles, 31
orthology, 25
out-of-body experiences, 15, 47–48
overvalued ideas, 35

Pais, Abraham, 60
paraphiers and paraphrands, 6, 16, 38, 56–57. *see also* metaphor
Park Keum Chul, 146
Pauli, Wolfgang, 66, 72
Pearson, Karl, 25, 59
Penfield, Wilder, 71–72
Penrose, Roger, 68–69
perception, supersensory, 72–73, 90–94
Percival, Ian, 120
Pettinato, Giovanni, 164–165
Phaedrus (Plato), 32
"Physics and Reality" (Einstein), 59
physio-kundalini syndrome, 171
Piaget, Jean, 55–56
pineal gland, 73, 81, 152–153, 183
Planck, Max, 59, 66, 120
Plato, 32
Platonism, 68
plexuses, 133
poetry as the stuff of consciousness, 5–6
Poincaré, Henri, 14
Ponce, Charles, 74, 131
Popper, Karl, 170
Porter Sargent Publishers, Inc., 81–82
Posner molecules, 69
possession (spiritual), 31–32
Poulin, Melissa Reeser, 56
prayer, 22, 176
pre-conscious hypostases, 23–24
Pribam, Karl, 69
Primo microcells, 148
Primo vascular system, 147
prisca sapienta (Newton), 123–124

Project for a Scientific Psychology (Freud), 111–112
prophets and prophecy, 25–30, 106, 159–161, 167–169, 171, 181
protoplasm, consciousness as property of, 7
Proverbs (Bible), 160–161
Psalms, 30, 123, 164
psyche (Greek word), 17, 24, 51–52, 56
psychedelics, 153, 154
psychoanalysis, 33–34, 114
psychology, 111–112
psychophysical parallelism, 65–66

Qi (Chinese medicine), 3, 73, 74, 122, 144, 171
Qi-gong psychotic reaction, 171
quantum mechanics
  in basis of consciousness, 57–60, 63–66, 68–72, 118–120, 129–130
  Copenhagen Interpretation, 58–59, 67
  direct consciousness of, 72–73, 90–94
  entanglement, 61–62
  FAPP (for all practical purposes), 67–69
  and mysticism, 64–67, 72–75, 178
  and Reissner's fiber, 2–3, 90–94, 118–120, 172–180, 182–184
  superconductivity, 118–119
  wave function, 65–66, 68, 70–71
quantum orthodoxy, 58–61, 65, 67
Quine, Willard, 49

Radin, Dean, 71
Rakic, Pasko, 85, 156
Raziel, Book of, 122, 126
reasoning, Jaynes's assessment of, 14
Reissner, Ernst, 76
Reissner's cells, 78
Reissner's fiber
  in acupuncture, 144–148
  anatomy of, 76–77, 81, 82, 85–87
  body regulation potential, 128–129, 176
  in circumneurocelic sensory system, 88–93

discovery and early studies, 76–79
evolution, 2–4, 98, 172–173
experiments, 84–85, 147–148, 157–158
in humans, 86–93, 150, 171–176
in Kabbalah, 122–123, 130–132
in *kundalini*, 133–136, 140–143
"monstrous moonshine", 179
Porter Sargent's studies, 79–82
post-Sargent studies, 82–87
in quantum systems, 2–3, 90–94, 118–120, 172–180, 182–184
regeneration, 4, 174–175
telephone line metaphor, 113–114
Wile's research, 153–158
Wile's unified neurocosmology, 172
relativity, 59, 96–97, 99
Rele, Vasant, 135–141, 156
religion. *see* scientists on religion
reticular activating system, 10
Roerich, Nicholas, 142
Rolland, Romain, 115
Rosen, Nathan, 62
Roth, Willard, 156

Sages of Shklov, 131
Samuel (prophet), 28–29
Samuel, Herbert L., 100
sanals (Primo microcells), 145, 148
Sargent, Porter, 79–82, 157
Saul, King of Israel, 28–29
schizophrenia, 5, 18, 29, 32–34, 49, 170–171
Schneersohn, Shalom Dov-Ber, 113–114
Scholem, Gershon, 131
Schrödinger, Erwin, 46, 60, 66, 72, 91
Schrödinger equation, 60, 64, 65–66, 90
Schrödinger's cat, 65, 91
scientists on religion
  Cantor, 99–100
  Einstein, 98–99, 100–104, 106–111, 120–121, 184
  Freud, 111–117

Jaynes, 33–34, 94–95, 174
Newton, 108–109
Spinoza, 104–107
SCO. *see* subcommissural organ
Secret of the Heavens (Swedenborg), 78
Sefer HaTemunah (Kabbalah), 122–123
self-reference and strange loops, 37, 44, 45, 52
sense impressions, 97–98
Sephirot (Kabbalah), 3, 73–74, 106, 122–123, 127–128, 130–131
Sergienko, Alexander, 178
sexuality, 114, 115, 130–131
Shalom, Abraham, 105
Shekinah (Kabbalah), 74, 115
Shimon bar Yochai, 129–130
Shroud of Turin, 129
singularity, initial, 2, 99, 123, 125, 172, 173
Smith, Edwin, 150
Snell, Bruno, 51–53
Soh Kwang Sop, 146–147
Solomon, King of Israel, 160, 161
Solovine, Maurice, 101
soma (Greek word), 24
Sommerfield, Arnold, 118
Sperry, Roger, 71
Spinoza, Baruch, 101, 104–107, 109–110, 120
spondins, 85–86, 179
Stapp, Henry, 68
stelae, 21, 162–163
Stieda, Ludwig, 77, 79
Stojkovic, Stephan, 180
strange loops, 37, 44, 45 52
Strauss, Ernst, 61
Studies on Hysteria (Freud and Breuer), 112
Studnicka, F.K., 79, 80, 83
subcommissural organ (SCO)
  experiments, 171
  function, 86, 155
  in hydrocephalus, 87
  origin of Reissner's fiber, 79–81, 83–85, 183
  outside the blood-brain barrier,

156
regression, 87–88
subtle anatomy
  in acupuncture, 144–148
  defined, 73–74
  in Kabbalah, 74, 114, 117, 126–132
  in near-death experiences, 87
  physical basis, 74
  Wile's neurocosmology, 3, 172
  Wile's studies, 148–158
  in yoga, 132–144
"Sunlight" (Heaney), 56
superconductivity, 118–119
supersensory perception, 72–73, 90–94
Sushumna nadi (yoga), 133–144, 146, 154
Susskind, Leonard, 124
Sutras of Pantajali, 132
Swedenborg, Emanuel, 77–78, 151

Tabernacle (Torah), 126–127
Talmud, 127, 128, 131, 160, 163, 181
Tantric yoga, 134–135, 140–143
The Tao of Physics, 72
Taoism, 73, 144, 148
Tel Dan Stele, 163
thalamus, 152
Theogony (Hesiod), 50
A Theologico-Political Treatise (Spinoza), 109–110
thinking, Jaynes's assessment of, 12–13
Thorn, Kip, 93
thumos (Greek word), 23, 49, 51–52
Tipler, Frank, 129
Tolstoy, Leo, 154–155
Torah, 110, 126–127
transcendental ego, 45–46, 57. *see also* analog "I"
Tretjakov, Dimitri, 88
Tukulti-Ninurta I (King of Assyria), 22

Umezawa, Hiroomi, 68
understanding, Jaynes's assessment of, 15–16
universal determinism, 101
Upanishads, 30

vagus nerve, 135–140
Vajra nadi (yoga), 134, 135, 154
Vatay, Gabor, 120
Vedas, 30
Vedic gods, 139–140
Vedic Gods as Figures of Biology (Rele), 139–140
verbal association experiment, 13
Vilkov, Grigory, 171
Vilna Gaon, 131
Vishnu-devananda, 142
visual hallucinations, 27, 166
Vital, Chayim, 115, 130
Vivekananda, 132–134, 142
voluntary control of body regulation, 136–137, 176
Von Neumann, John, 65–66

Wachter, Georg, 105
Wallace, Alfred Russel, 8, 126
Watson, John B., 9
Watt, H.J., 13
weight-judging experiment, 13, 43
Wernicke, Carl, 35
Wernicke's area, 18, 39, 47
Whitehead, Alfred North, 6
Wigner, Eugene, 66
Wile, Lawrence
  with C. Loeser, 85, 148–158
  on near-death experiences, 87
  on *Sushumna nadi* and *Sephirot*, 131
  unified neurocosmology, 3–4, 172
  zebrafish experiments, 177–179
"Wile's hormone", 153–154
Willis, Thomas, 151
Witten, Edward, 179, 183–184
Wittgenstein, Ludwig, 45
Woodroffe, Sir John, 134–135
Woollam, D.H.M., 86–87
Work and Days (Hesiod), 49
Wright, John Henry, 132

Yahuda, Abraham, 108
Yahweh, 26, 163–165, 166, 167
Yisrael Baal Shem Tov, 131
yoga. *see also kundalini*
  methods and exercises, 138–139, 175

"subtle anatomy" in, 132–140
Tantra, 134–135, 140–143
Yogananda, Paramahansa, 142, 154

zebrafish experiments, 177–179
Zechariah (prophet), 30, 169

Zedekiah, King of Judah, 168–169
Zeno effect, 68
zero point fluctuations, 120
Zhdanova, Irina, 179
Zohar, 110, 115

www.ingramcontent.com/pod-product-compliance
Lightning Source LLC
Chambersburg PA
CBHW081216230426
43666CB00015B/2750